From Chronically Stressed to Fully Blessed

A Faith-Filled Functional
Medicine Approach to
Breaking Free from
Stress and Overwhelm

GRETCHEN REIS, MD

DISCLAIMERS

To protect privacy, some names in this book have been changed.

This book is not intended as a substitute for the medical advice of a physician. The reader should regularly consult a physician in matters relating to his or her health and particularly with respect to any symptoms that may require diagnosis or medical attention. Statements regarding products have not been evaluated by the Food and Drug Administration. Any products or treatment regimens are not intended to diagnose, treat, cure or prevent any disease. If you are pregnant, nursing, taking medication, or have a medical condition, consult your health care professional before using any products based on this content.

The information in this book is for general health knowledge only. Results of medical treatments vary, and the author assumes no liability or responsibility for any actions taken by the reader or any outcomes thereof.

*"And God is able to make all grace abound to you,
so that having all sufficiency in all things at all times,
you may abound in every good work."*

2 Corinthians 9:8 ESV

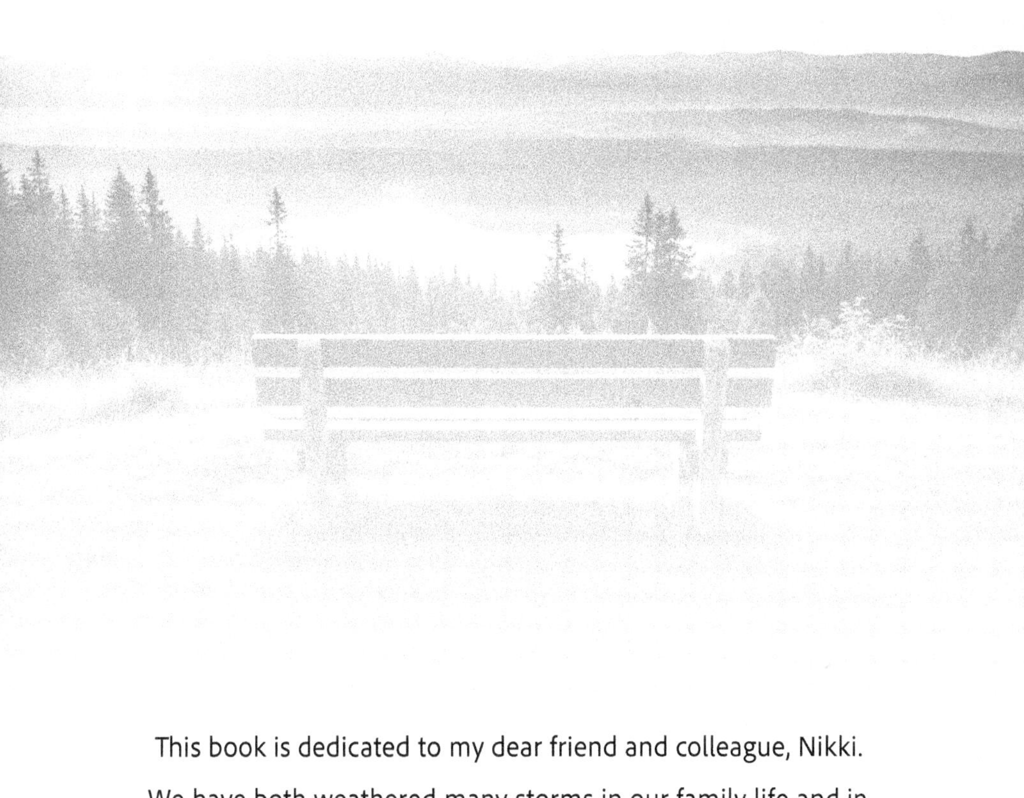

This book is dedicated to my dear friend and colleague, Nikki.

We have both weathered many storms in our family life and in
our careers, but we constantly remind each other that
"I may be in the storm, but the storm is not in me . . . Jesus is."

TABLE OF CONTENTS

Introduction:
Change Your Perspective

Stress is inescapable, and everyone experiences it to some degree. There are seasons of high stress, and there are seasons of rest and ease. That's just life. In recent years, though, the world seems to be under more stress, as manifestations of evil become ever more apparent. We see it in crime on the streets, power hungry leaders, economic hardship, and spiritual persecution. The power of darkness is more out in the open, and this reflects itself in our lives in a myriad of ways.

I want to start off by challenging you to reconsider how you view stress. It's not black and white like good versus evil. Stress is a powerful force that can draw us closer to God and His purpose for our lives. It can adjust our attitudes. It can help us focus on what's *important*, not just what's *urgent*. It is not just something bad that threatens to consume your life and your emotions. It is an incredible opportunity for growth! Yes, it hurts, it's hard, and we hate it. But I want you to keep an open mind to the possibilities that lie within the discomfort.

These possibilities start to be seen by digging in to understand stress. Here we will talk about why and how we experience stress, and then we will look at how harmful it is to the human body. Stress can affect your mental health, your physical health, and your spiritual health. Beyond all that, it affects everyone around you. We will also look at all the ways we can resist the negative effects of stress, and then we will consider some of the positive changes we can see when stress is handled appropriately. You might learn to embrace stress as your perspective changes. Well, you can at least embrace the opportunity it presents! With training, you can see it as an opportunity and respond in a constructive, positive way. You will reap the reward of growth and blessing on the other side if you persevere. It's called overcoming!

No Magic Pill for Stress

You know the old saying about the more you learn, the more you realize how much you don't know? That definitely applies to medicine. The more I have learned over the past twenty-five years in practice, the more I realize how much I still don't understand or know how to fix in patients. Some medical conditions are unexplained and difficult to treat, and all we can do is to try to reduce symptoms. We don't have a cure for everything, which is very frustrating. Cancer, heart disease, dementia, and many other chronic diseases simply don't have easy cures. We try our best and have come a long way with treatment, but all too often, the disease wins out.

Stress is like that, too. There is no magic pill to make it go away. Sometimes you manage it and reduce the effect it has on you. I have experienced a lot of stress in my life. I'll share some of it as we go, but with all I've been through, I feel like I should have some answers by now, some wise insight, or a sure-fire way of coping with stress. But I don't. Even though I have walked through a lot of hard times, I sometimes feel like I'm right back where I started. Frustrated, disappointed, and tired. This is not a book with all the answers or a magic cure. We each walk through our own valleys and "work out your own salvation with fear and trembling" (Philippians 2:12). Our journey is unique to God's purpose in our lives. I hope to give you tools to understand what is happening with your emotions and your body. Once you realize what is happening and appreciate how serious it is, you can start to proactively manage it in a positive way.

Response to Stress

When we are stressed, we usually spin down into a hole of negative emotions and feel sorry for ourselves. We withdraw from other people and are not as giving or loving. Some people live in a constant state of self-pity, oblivious to what other people are going through. It's hard for God to use us to bless others when we are in this state. Most of us stay in this hole of negative emotions until the stress subsides, then we get back to normal. We are often not even aware of how we have treated others.

But it doesn't need to be this way. The Serenity Prayer tells us, "God grant me the serenity to accept the things I cannot change; Courage to change the things I can; And wisdom to know the difference." [1]

You can choose to be passive and wallow in your stress, or you can be active in managing it. How? You can learn to ask yourself: "What can I change, and what can't I change?" There is tremendous power in accepting the things you cannot change and changing your response to those things.

When a stressful situation comes into your life, it usually doesn't seem fair. I often don't understand why I am suffering. But that's when you need faith: trusting that He is using it for good. Paul tells us, "All things work together for good to those who love God, to those who are the called according to His purpose" (Romans 8:28). The challenge is to allow God to move through you, and then purposefully choose your responses.

There is a lot you can do to reduce the effect stress has on your body and your mind. I want to show you how powerful these tools can be. God does not want you sick from your stress! He wants to use the stress to form you into a better person. Diamonds are made under tremendous pressure. My challenge to you starts right now: start thinking about stress as a positive process that is making you more like God. Although it is painful, it can be good for you. It shapes your character and your faith. It is what God uses to make you more useful to him. Isn't that what the Christian life is about?

Selye and Sapolsky

What exactly is stress? Stress is defined as "a specific response by the body to a stimulus, as fear or pain, that disturbs or interferes with the normal physiological equilibrium of an organism."[2] The word "stress" causes an immediate negative emotional reaction in most people. We simply assume stress is bad, but there are many stresses that are good. Spring training makes a football team ready when the season opens. A deadline for the project at work makes you productive and efficient. A tight budget causes you to cook at home instead of eating out. A final exam pushes you to study and learn the material. These stressors force us to behave in a mature, responsible way instead of just doing what our flesh wants. But other stressors can be hard on us emotionally. Because we don't see the reason for them, there is no goal or sense of accomplishment. When a loved one dies, your roof needs to be replaced, or you are let go at work, it can be hard to see the good. If we see the reason, we will work hard to achieve the goal. But when something just seems like there is no good at all in it, it can be very hard to cope with. This type of stress is what we need to look at. If we can find ways to cope and find some good in it, life becomes much easier.

Dr. Hans Selye was an endocrinologist who started studying the stress response in the 1930s. He wrote a groundbreaking book, *The Stress of Life,* in 1956.[3] In it, he describes three phases of the stress response: alarm, adaptation, and exhaustion. His work explained a great deal about the physiological changes that occur with acute or ongoing stress.

Robert Sapolsky is a neuroendocrinology expert who wrote another great book on stress, *Why Zebras Don't Get Ulcers.* This book explains that in general, when animals experience stress, it is quick to occur and then quick to resolve.[4] The zebra being chased by a lion either escapes and then goes to munch on grass somewhere else, or it is killed and the game is over. Short-term stress serves a real purpose: to keep you alive. After the stress, an animal goes right back to a calm state, in some ways forgetting what just happened. But when humans suffer ongoing, chronic stress, the constantly-elevated stress hormones eventually wear down the entire body and disease results. Zebras don't get ulcers, gray hair, high blood pressure, or dementia. People do.

Stress is a Slow Killer

In my thirty-plus years as a physician, I can absolutely attest to the fact that stress is a factor in many, if not most, chronic diseases and in virtually all mental health conditions. Stress contributes to cancer, heart disease, arthritis, and even dementia. If you include poor lifestyle choices made because of being stressed, the list is virtually endless. My husband, Bill, is a life and nutrition coach. He believes that if someone gets their diet and lifestyle habits optimized and learns how to manage stress, they can avoid many diseases. Many times, I have been unable to help patients because they refused to deal with their stress and their unhealthy lifestyle choices. Prescriptions can't fix their choices . . . they only are a temporary help. I challenge my patients every day to put me out of business. But alas, stress becomes a seemingly insurmountable challenge and people get stuck in destructive habits.

While you are probably thinking you understand you are stressed, what you don't know is all the damage that's happening to your body. This is a silent epidemic, wreaking havoc in your body, and you have no idea how destructive it is. We want to think it's just a mental or emotional effect, but it's way beyond that . . . stress can lead to permanent damage to your gastrointestinal system, your brain, and the rest of your body. It can even cause cancer and heart disease, which can kill you.

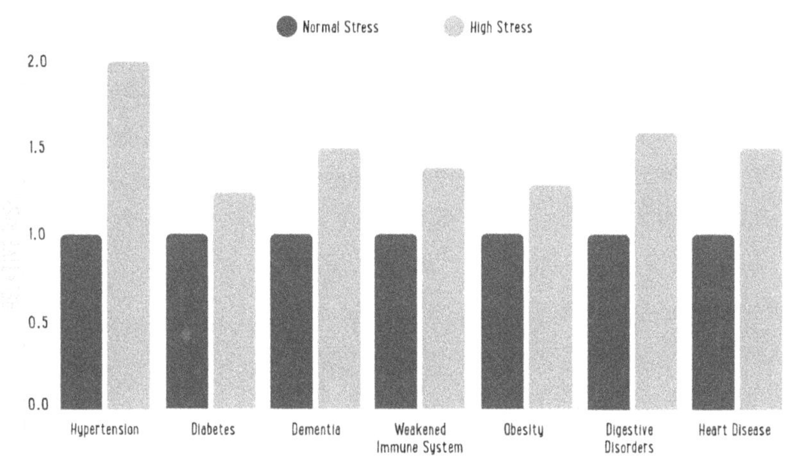

hypertension – 2x
diabetes – 1.25x
dementia – 1.5x
weakened immune system – 1.4x
obesity – 1.3 x
digestive disorders – 1.6x
heart disease – 1.5x

That's the depressing news. For now, it's probably good that it scares you a bit. My hope is that you will take stress seriously and do something about it. While we have no control over what happens to us, we have total control over our reaction to it!

Good News About Stress

We all intuitively know when a situation isn't working well and isn't what it could be. The good news for Christians is that this proves our spirit is longing for Heaven! We know deep down we were designed to live in peace with loving relationships and to have our needs met. Adam and Eve experienced that in the garden before they messed it up. But living in a fallen world means that things often are annoying, frustrating, or maddening because they just aren't right. Our longing for stress resolution is really the longing our spirit has to be with God and to be fully immersed in His peace. When we get to Heaven, all will be right, and our stress will be gone. In the meantime, live in God's grace to be strong and do all you can. This book is to educate you and inspire you to do the best you can. This promise is ours: "Therefore take up the whole armor of God, that you may be able to withstand in the evil day, and having done all, to stand" (Ephesians 6:13).

Your job is to do what you can do. God's job is to do all the rest . . . that's His grace at work. Evangelist Jerry Savelle loved to talk about playing checkers with God. While playing, it sometimes is clearly our turn. God is waiting for us to make a move. He sits patiently, waiting for us to obey what He would have us do. After you do your part, it's His turn. We wait patiently in faith for Him to move. We need to know Him well enough that we know whose turn it is in any situation.

God is the one that can heal a broken marriage or straighten out a troubled teen. He can give you a new job or a raise. If you've done all you know God wants you to do, let God take His turn. What we do is so small compared to what God does! Be like John the Baptist when he said, "He must increase, but I must decrease" (John 3:30). His works are much greater than anything we can do. God's work is perfect and powerful.

Imperfect Can Be Perfect

Remember the goal is not to be stress-free, but to be used by God for good. When we are depressed, frantic, or in a brain fog, we are self-centered on our own problems and are not looking for ways we can bring hope and joy to others. God allows hardships and trials as a means to an end. We can choose to get depressed and angry at the situation, or we can choose to embrace the challenge and view it as an opportunity for the power of God to move. Here's a key concept that you know but may often forget: you can't change much of anything that is happening to you, but you have full control over how you react. Now that is empowering.

We can embrace imperfection, because it is perfect from God's perspective. Say what? It is God's will (perfect) to be in a state of imperfection. Take a minute to think about that. Paul said, "For I have learned in whatever state I am, to be content" (Philippians 4:11). Life is just not ever going to be perfect. You may have moments lying on a sunny beach on vacation that feel close to perfect. But sooner or later, the rain comes or you go home and back to work. If you're relying on the absence of stress to be happy and usable by God, you'll be disappointed much of the time, and God won't be able to use you. How sad is the thought that God had plans to use you, but you were so self-centered that He passed you by and couldn't use you? What a waste.

There is so much freedom in letting go. Many of us, especially women, like to be in control. We like our homes beautiful and clean, we manage complicated family schedules, and we just keep going all day long. But of course, most of us struggle to keep our homes free of clutter, and the dishes sometimes sit on the counter too long. We just can't do everything all the time. We often beat ourselves up with critical self-talk. Imagine a CEO who thinks they can do everything without an assistant. They try to take all their calls, schedule meetings, type and print reports, arrange travel, and implement projects all on their own. Then when they are stressed and make a mistake on something, they berate themselves. Sound ridiculous? It sure is, because a good assistant can make the CEO's life so much smoother and effective. You trying to do everything without any time for yourself and without God is just as stressful and ineffective.

For those of you who are now saying "but there is just so much I have to do in my day!"—I get it. I really do! But when you actually take time to assess your time management and your goals, you may find some wasted time (social media, TV) or activities that maybe aren't so crucial that you can eliminate. It's okay to not get *everything* done in a day. The task will be there tomorrow. When you let go of needing to be in control and you accept imperfection, peace flows in and God can fill your life. The adage to "let go and let God" is true. When there is a hole in our life, let God fill it by letting go. Remember that God's still in control . . . we don't have to be!

Let's dive in, and first, figure out why we are so stressed.

CHAPTER 1

Ubiquity of Stress

Why are we so stressed? Compared to the lives our grandparents and great-grandparents had, we have it easy. We have machines that wash and dry our clothes, a dishwasher that cleans a kitchen's worth of dirty dishes, and we have clean, hot running water to bathe in all the time. We have an abundance of food and comfortable beds. We drive and fly everywhere in very little time. We have so much more than people who lived only one hundred years ago. We should be relaxed and enjoying all the free time we have from not having to work as hard. But it doesn't seem to work that way.

Consider the advances we have made with technology. If you're my age or older, you remember corded phones hanging in the kitchen and busy signals. You remember looking things up in the library or in your *Encyclopedia Brittanica.* You used classified ads and the yellow pages to find resources. Now we can look something up on our phones or even ask the smart speaker in the house, and you instantly have your answer. We bank online, order food online, and take pictures and send them to others instantly.

You would think our grandparents and great-grandparents would have been miserable because of how hard life was. But they weren't—that's just how life was. They knew hard work, disease, and death were a part of life. I would argue that people were more content with life then than many of us now, because they did not expect their lives to be perfect. They appreciated the good things in life so much more than we often do.

Happiness and contentment are highly subjective, and one of the themes of this book is learning that you have a lot of control over both. You don't need to be a passive victim of stressful circumstances. You can choose your reaction. My grandmother had a son who was deaf and died when he was only five years old. She then lost her husband to cancer when he was only in his forties. She chose to walk in strength and moved through her grief, living a good life all the rest of her days.

Contentment and satisfaction are things we want to achieve. When we are stressed, we feel discontent and are not satisfied. I would argue that there is a big difference between contentment and satisfaction. One way to describe contentment is to experience ease of mind. This is the state of calm, peace, and not worrying. I liken it to being totally okay with where you are right now. Maybe not forever, but in this moment, you're okay.

Satisfaction is a state of fulfillment, though, which is a longer-term result. When a project is completed, you are satisfied. However, during the process, you can be content with your progress without being fully satisfied. One of the secrets of stress management is to be content with your current position, even if you aren't satisfied with the results yet.

Why are we so highly stressed, dissatisfied, and discontent? We should have so much extra time now! Why aren't we relaxed with a lot of extra time on our hands? There are a lot of opinions on this, and a lot of reasons that are unique to each person. The answer usually lies in the fact that we choose to be stressed, because we refuse to relax. We fill our time with more stuff and more activities, increasing our stressors. More is not always good and there is much truth in saying, "Less is best."

Schedules

If you have a child that plays sports, you know exactly what it's like for huge chunks of your weekly schedule to be filled with practices and games. For parents, that added responsibility seems to fill up our days as soon as the sports season begins. If you get a break between basketball season and track season, you may savor that time knowing that when practices begin again, you'll go back to spending a lot of time in the car or at the field. Add in driving your kids to and from school, and you may feel like you live in your car!

For women, our modern era hasn't always worked out so well. Although having a little house on the prairie in the 1800s sure wasn't easy, the wife never had to go work a job for eight hours and then come home, cook, do laundry, and help with homework. She had time during the day to maintain her household. The modern woman has so many career opportunities available that simply weren't an option decades ago. We have been liberated, right? But with all the advances of modern life, why aren't we happy? With the rapid pace of our society, we have sped up, too.

Men also have busier schedules. Work may extend beyond the typical workday, and some men are stay-at-home dads which can be much more work than some office jobs. Some homeschool their kids. Add on workouts at the gym, the occasional social get-together, and kids' activities, and men's schedules are just as busy as women's.

It's not just the adults that are busy. Kids nowadays are also busier. When I was growing up in the 1970s, most of us kids in the neighborhood did a little homework after school, then ran around and played the rest of the day. It was a long time ago, but I rarely had homework to do after dinner. We got exercise and were learning social skills just roaming the neighborhood as a group. I don't remember any of my friends being involved in any activities other than scouting in elementary school. We didn't have a lot of sports teams and formal activities when I grew up.

Often these activities create so much stress in parents and kids that they cause fatigue, anxiety, and depression. If you believe that your child must have a list of accomplishments a mile long to get into college, it's not true! Some of the most elite schools that require detailed resumes to get into are ones that promote values that are opposite the Christian worldview. You really don't want to send your child there. You can get a good education at a community or state college, and here's a shocking thought: not everyone needs to go to college! Don't sign your son up for basketball when he's ten years old just because you think he needs it to go to an Ivy League school. Only do it if he truly enjoys basketball.

Ask yourself this: When was the last time you had four hours with nothing scheduled? What did you do with your time? Did you catch up on chores or errands, or did you just sit and do nothing? If I asked you to sit and do nothing for four hours, what would your reaction be? Mine would be, "You're kidding, right? I can't just sit and do nothing!" This is probably why so many of us turn on the TV when we have nothing to do. While that isn't inherently bad, if you watch too much TV, you may not be relaxing in a good way. Tuning out the world works for a short time, but it's much better to truly relax and cultivate relationships. This moves you forward and increases your stress resilience.

When you think about boredom, do you think of it as something bad? I challenge you to cultivate boredom. It is so good for us to have blocks of time with no responsibilities. I love to take time on a summer evening to sit out on my back deck and read a book. I may take my dog for an extra walk on Saturdays in the fall, and then I'll spend some time watching football with my family. I think we all enjoy just sitting in a comfortable chair on the beach and doing nothing.

When I was young, I kept a diary. I have obsessive-compulsive disorder (OCD) tendencies, which pushed me to make an entry every day. I laugh now when I remember how often I wrote, "Today was a nothing day." (I just couldn't leave a page blank!) Don't you just love a delicious Sunday afternoon and evening when you have nowhere to go and nothing to do? This time is a gift from God, and we need to seek it out and thoroughly enjoy it. Avoid over scheduling yourself and adding to your stress. The Psalms remind us, "This is the day that the Lord has made; We will rejoice and be glad in it" (Psalm 118:24). It's more than okay to fully enjoy times of relaxation. They create joy, which is exactly what God wants for us!

Beware the trap of being too busy. You just might be making yourself miserable and sick.

Change in Family Structure

Another reason why many people are so stressed is the increase in single-parent homes. Most sociologists and historians will tell you that societies that embrace the traditional family structure are more successful and thrive. There are many reasons for this, but, overall, research data indicates the biblical view of family and marriage is the healthiest model.

Studies have linked single parent homes with higher rates of stress and depression. Socioeconomic factors also correlate with depression, so being a single parent without sufficient economic resources is even more stressful on the family.[5] Children raised without a mother and father have higher rates of depression, anxiety, poor school performance and substance use.[6] Children whose parents have divorced have reduced school performance, more mental health issues, more learning disabilities, and more sickness.[7]

In our modern world, people get divorced at an alarming rate. The divorce rate before World War II was under two per one thousand people. It then increased to a high of around five per one thousand people in the 1980s.[8] It has decreased somewhat since then, thankfully. But it is still true that about half of all marriages in the US will end in divorce or separation. Divorce is one of those life-changing stressors that leaves an impact for a long time afterward.

Babies born to unwed mothers have skyrocketed in the past twenty years. According to the Annie E. Casey Foundation (Kids Count Data Center), data from 2019 shows that 64 percent of black children are being raised by a single parent.[9] Marriage has decreased so much that a majority of black women are raising their children alone. Rates of single parenting in Native American and Hispanic culture are also much higher than in Caucasians. There are many contributing factors to these statistics, but suffice it to say, a significant portion of the younger generation are growing up without both a mother and a father present in the home.

We generally think of women as being single parents, but single men also struggle to raise children. Years ago, one of my cousins had two beautiful young daughters, and his wife just simply walked out one day and left, never to be seen again. This was a long time ago, and the girls have turned out to be amazing women and mothers themselves, but we all were in complete shock. This kind of abandonment brings grief and stress. Death of a parent is also devastating to families.

No matter which parent leaves and why, it's enormously stressful. When you work full time and then come home and take care of children, your day is going to be long and intense. You don't have a partner to share the workload with. This takes a toll and is a major contributor to stress.

Another family stress is dysfunction. I cannot tell you how many times I've seen a patient who tearfully tells me all about their crazy family members and the strife they cause. Some of the worst stories are the ones about siblings who fight after the parent dies. They argue about the estate and get lawyers, creating so much emotional pain all around. The other situation is the mother who guilts her children into doing things. One of my favorite television shows used to be *Everybody Loves Raymond*. The mother in this show was played brilliantly by Doris Roberts. She was an expert in manipulating everyone in her family by using guilt. It was a funny take on a common behavior that isn't so funny in real life.

If you have family members who manipulate others with their emotional reactions and behavior, stress is inevitable. You can't change that person's behavior, and it's very difficult to change who your family is. This issue, especially if codependency is involved, requires thorough analysis and a careful change in your responses. Find a good counselor to walk with you through this. You simply cannot make other people happy, and you aren't responsible for their emotions. Take the high ground, but do not allow yourself to get pulled down. Walk above the fray as much as possible.

Less Community

Stress is also increased dramatically when you are in social isolation from others. We are designed to need, support, and live life with others. That's how God wants it to be. God said, "It is not good that man should be alone; I will make him a helper comparable to him" (Genesis 2:18). This applies not just to men and how much they need women (*I can hear you laughing*) but also for us women. We need each other!

Marriage is a covenant we make to each other and provides stability in our faith, our family, and our community. If you are having relationship issues in your marriage, this will be a great source of stress, and I encourage you to seek godly counseling. You will need someone to help you define the issues and help you both work toward healing. Having a loving partner can either make or break you in your journey. Don't let the enemy rob you of the joy of having someone on your side who loves you and supports you.

We also need community connection with other family members, neighbors, friends and other church members. Modern society has made community connection much more difficult than it used to be. I remember running all over the neighborhood growing up and we knew our neighbors. We would walk around the block and see who else was out so we could say hi or even chat.

Today we often live in subdivisions behind closed and air-conditioned doors and don't meet our neighbors like we should. Even if you live in the city with a front porch, people just aren't out as much to connect like they have been in previous generations. People walk down the street with their eyes glued to their phone. Folks run or walk their dog with headphones on. We run on the treadmill at the gym with earbuds. We have gone from Mayberry on *The Andy Griffith Show* to walking around like robots.

Wherever you live, make an effort to connect with others in a community. This may be your physical neighborhood, your church or synagogue, a networking group, a pickleball group or a hobby you participate in. Our church has worked very hard the past few years to build up home groups we call *life groups*. I like this name because community is life. When we get together and share our struggles and frustrations, our successes and our dreams, we are drawn together in God's love and strengthened. Just knowing I have a friend praying for my problem gives me strength. Counselors will tell you how therapeutic talking about your problem can be. Then if you add compassionate friends who will come by your side and walk through the problem with you, you will be strong and capable of emerging on the other side so much better for it. Cultivate community around you. Your health needs it!

Less Exercise

We all know that exercise is good for us, but many of us just don't do it enough. It clearly is good for your brain health, heart health, weight, and your energy. But did you know that exercise is one of the best stress busters there is?

I like to say that if more people knew how powerful hormone balance, nutrition, and regular exercise are, we would slash rates of chronic disease and people would be so much happier. Pharmaceutical sales would drop, and some specialists would be out of a job. That wouldn't be so good for the medical industrial complex. But it would be miraculous for all those healthy people!

I'm sure you have used all the same excuses I have about exercise: I don't have time. It's too far to go to the gym. It's too hot or too cold outside. I can't afford it. I don't like to work out alone. I don't like taking classes. I hate weights. I hate cardio. My dog ate my homework. *(Well, maybe not that one!)* Now certainly there are situations that are true reasons and not just excuses. In my case, I love to run, but I have a special needs son at home that has seizures and has limited ability to care for his own needs. When I'm at home with him, even though he is a young adult, I can't go running. If he had a seizure unattended, it could be very bad. But I can't use that as an excuse to never run. I have to be creative and simply can't run as often as I would like, but I don't give up.

If you're like me, you like to get your steps in. I remember getting a fitness watch years ago and tracking my steps, trying to get that 10,000 steps in every day. I wasn't always successful, but I did start parking a little farther back at the grocery store and I took the stairs more often. Sedentary jobs, especially working from home on a computer, are a big reason why we don't get as much exercise as our ancestors did. You absolutely need to get up from your desk frequently and walk around a little bit. Even better, go outside for five to ten minutes. Moving around in sunshine and fresh air can greatly reduce your stress!

One of the biggest benefits from exercise that you may not be aware of is that it reduces the impact that stress has on our bodies. In addition to building muscle and feeling a mental boost in energy and mood, exercise also acts as a buffer to the things that cortisol and inflammation can do. We'll go into the details in a later chapter, but exercise prevents the damage that stress can do to your body.

Many of us don't have as much time to exercise as we would like. You might also believe that you have to work out five days a week, so you may feel like lesser amounts of exercise are not worth it. That is not true! Even being a weekend warrior, with physical activity on Saturday and Sunday, will help your health more than being sedentary. Get outside and work around the house on weekends. Just doing some yard work or gardening will give you exercise, as well as sunshine and fresh air. Consider taking up a hobby. It could be refinishing old furniture, building model train sets, or disc golf. Pretty much anything that isn't sitting around will work and can be fun!

You may also feel like you need to work out strenuously for it to count. Some of my patients are over-exercisers. They do boot-camp-style workouts, flipping tires and doing strenuous exercises for an hour or more every day. Some women do this, mistakenly believing they will lose weight the more they work out. But it usually doesn't work. High intensity exercise will raise cortisol which can create physical issues and prevent weight loss. Sometimes the muscle you gain, along with the stress of the high intensity workout, makes you gain weight. The right balance with your exercise routine is important. The best exercise for stress relief consists of mild to moderate exertion, and it does not have to be for a long time. I encourage my patients to start with getting outside for a fifteen-minute walk. This one goal is more than enough to make your brain and moods more resistant to stress.

Long Days

When we lived in a rural county in Ohio, my drive to work was only seven minutes. I could leave the house at 8:45 a.m. and still see my first patient at nine. I loved it! When we moved to Charlotte, my drive to work was about forty-five minutes. That took a while to adjust to. Over the next few years with the rapid growth in the area, my commute home turned into an hour or more. The length of my workday started contributing to my stress load. I had no time in the morning for myself, and I didn't get home until far later than I liked. It was not fun.

When we had the opportunity to relocate my office, we found the perfect location much closer to where we live. My drive is now around thirty minutes, so I have a little more time in the morning and evening. While most of you probably can't easily change where you live or work, if you have a long commute, please realize that it may be affecting you. If you commonly stop at a store or two on your way home from work—reducing your time with your family in the evening—consider what you can put off until another time or delegate to someone else. Getting home a little earlier and sharing dinner with your family is much better for your emotional stress than crossing off a few items on your to do list.

Make a purposeful decision about how you will use the time of your commute. You can grumble about traffic, slow drivers, construction or the weather, making yourself miserable. But you don't have to! Once again, you can't change your circumstance, but you can change your reaction to it. Use that time to listen to relaxing music or listen to a podcast or even preaching. Try to avoid listening to work-related topics, though. Leave work at work and fill your brain with something that is relaxing, motivating or inspirational. Make it your time to talk to God and focus on what God wants you to do and be. Then when you get to work in the morning or back home in the evening, you are calm and focused for the next part of your day.

Less Relaxing in the Evening

Most of us need to learn to slow down. We also need to learn to leave work at work and be home when at home. The line between work and home has become very blurred in the era of email and cell phones. Now that so many jobs have shifted to virtual work from home, it's even worse than ever. Many employees feel the need to monitor and respond to emails and texts in the evening. I admit I am old school, but I just don't understand this! I think it's important to work hard when you're working and stop for a break when you're not. When you mix in work tasks with your evening with your family, your efforts on either front are diluted. You will be distracted and not fully engaged. Then you will also feel like you are working all day long, and that contributes to stress. For years I was in a solo primary care practice, and I was on call for emergencies twenty-four seven. Patients called when they had an emergency, so it was truly necessary, but it was intense.

I have never understood why bosses feel the need to email or call employees after the workday ends. If it's not an emergency, it can wait until the next day. If you have a boss like that, I urge you to have a discussion with him or her. The next thing you can do is simply to not check your email in the evening. Or here's a wild and crazy idea: take your email off your phone. It's amazing how effective that is! It's just too easy to check your email or social media on your phone while you are watching television with your family. *Don't do it!* When you take all that stuff off your phone, your phone is much less distracting.

My husband has been telling me for over twenty years that I need to learn to relax. It's hard when the number of things to do is over-whelming and you feel like you have so little time, but relaxing is still important. When I hear my patients say they work all day and then take children to activities and go through a drive through, getting home at eight or nine at night, I get tired just imagining that schedule every day. Most of us run out of energy if we don't pace ourselves and learn to say no. Our bodies are designed to work during daylight and rest after dark. We can work longer days more easily in summer, but in winter, we are hardwired to relax in the evening. Some societies still basically go to bed as soon as it's dark, even in winter. While you shouldn't stop everything and go to bed at six in January, I do believe you need some time of relaxation in the evening. I know someone who works three jobs to provide for her family and works seven days a week. She has three children and just doesn't get enough time with them. This is not good for her or them. We need to slow down!

I will confess, I wanted to write this book for several years before I finally did. I just kept saying, "I don't have time to write!" My husband is my best cheerleader but also challenges me regularly. He repeatedly provoked me back to writing when I let it slide for a while. He also makes me realize that I am not prioritizing my time correctly. I can be too focused on keeping the house tidy, doing dishes, taking care of the dog and the trash and all the other stuff that keeps most of us busy through the evening. He reminds me that I don't have to get all those things done. And I quickly realized taking time to write was a matter of properly prioritizing my time.

My husband and I have taught Dave Ramsey's course Financial Peace several times. If you haven't taken it, you really need to. Whether you are struggling financially or are wealthy, you will benefit from this course. The entire foundation of the course is taking control of your money. You tell your money where it's going by using a budget for everything. Most people don't use a budget, and their money just flies out of their account throughout the month and runs out before the month runs out. When you stick to a budget, you won't run out of money. You are in control. If you budget $100 for clothing and spend it, that's it for the month—the next weekend, you don't go to the mall. You are in now control of your money.

The same concept applies to our time. I am famous (*infamous*) for not leaving work on time. Anyone who has worked in a doctor's office knows that closing time is not leaving time. Messages and paperwork pile up during the day and often keep doctors and staff there until way past closing time. Because if you don't do it that day, the work accumulates. Back in the old days of paper charts, there was often a stack of charts about two feet high on my desk at 5:30 p.m., all with messages on them. We had to address all of them before leaving for the day, so it was virtually impossible to get out "on time." Nowadays the messages are all electronic, so it's a bit easier to address them bit by bit throughout the day, but you still never know how much work there is to do after the last patient leaves.

Well, I have been more convicted of this recently. If I tell my husband I'll leave the office by 5:30, I need to take control of my time and make it happen. Rarely is someone on the phone with a medical emergency at 5:29. My new objective is to set a realistic time to leave the office and then *do it*. The messages or busywork can wait one more day! There is a show on Fox News called "The Five." The last segment in their one-hour show is called "One More Thing." Each host has thirty seconds to talk about a lighthearted story. This segment is sometimes funny or heartwarming, so it is popular. Interestingly, the producers will absolutely cut them off when time runs out, so even they have limits.

Don't let *one-more-thing-ism* afflict you at work. We all have it sometimes. *One more call. One more email. One more stack of papers to file. One more document to edit and print.* One more suddenly turns into fifteen more, and boom! You're late. Don't allow *one-more-thing-ism* to afflict you in the evening around the house, either. Just say no.

I am, admittedly, a work in progress. Compulsive tendencies try to get me all the time. I sometimes believe the delusion that, if my to-do list is all checked off and my office and home are neat as a pin, then I will finally be able to relax, but not until all that is done. That is a lie. Let the tasks go and embrace imperfection. Take back control of your time, investing in what really matters. Time on the couch watching a home renovation show with your spouse. Playing a card game with your kids. Calling a friend or a relative. We need to manage our time and guard it from all the things that try to steal our time. They can wait.

Less Nothing Time

We need time to just do absolutely nothing productive! I have always been energized by doing things and crossing things off my list. My sister used to call me a workaholic growing up, because I didn't stop working. I realize now that finishing a task gives my brain a little hit of dopamine, which can be energizing and addicting. What was seemingly good for me when I was younger now causes me stress. Life is more complicated now, and I need more rest to stay healthy.

I have patients who have told me they can't sit and watch a movie—they are too restless. They can force themselves to watch a thirty-minute show with their spouse but even that is very difficult. If this is you, you can work on being more comfortable at rest.

I have worked hard to balance my activity with rest. Like I mentioned in the previous section, I try not to do any work in the evening. My resolution this year has been to not check my work email in the evenings. On weekends, I try to blend chores with fun. My husband usually goes out to breakfast Saturdays with his men's group from church. I try to get all my stuff done in the morning, and then we can relax the rest of the day. That way, if we watch football all afternoon and then a movie at night, I don't feel guilty, and I truly can relax knowing I already got something done in the morning.

There has been a lot of research done on mindfulness, yoga, and meditation. These are methods of pushing out extra thoughts and simply being in the moment with your environment. Think about it: when was the last time you sat in a chair and did nothing for ten minutes? Consider the times you sat on the beach, watching the waves, and truly saw and appreciated the majesty of God's creation. Or the times you sat around a campfire with family or friends, just thinking about life. Mindfulness requires stillness.

Prayer is a form of mindfulness and is essential for a passion-filled Christian life. If you think you're too busy to pray, then you flat out are too busy! You need to slow down and intentionally carve out time in your day for your mind to settle down and for all your worries to subside. We live our lives and our schedules like a snow globe constantly in motion. When we sit and get still, all the noise settles down, and we can see much more clearly.

We cannot truly know God unless *and until* we are still. The Psalmist writes, "Be still, and know that I am God: I will be exalted among the heathen, I will be exalted in the earth" (Psalm 46:10 KJV). The only way to truly know Him and hear His voice is to slow down and listen. Being still is hard for me, but I'm a lot better than I used to be. This section is misnamed, as "Nothing Time" is not nothing. It is a very powerful tool that God commands us to do, and He uses it to heal our anxious minds. "Nothing time" has the power to make everything possible!

ACEs (Increase Susceptibility to Stress)

We all vary in our response to stress. It fascinates me to see some of my patients literally losing sleep worrying about virtually nothing. Lisa has three children who cause her endless anxiety. One has an MBA and works in finance, one is in college, and one is still in high school. All of them are doing well, but she still worries about them all the time! She told me she calls her grown children every day, and if she doesn't talk to them, she gets anxious. Contrast that with Kristin, who lost her daughter to a drug overdose a few years ago. She is bright, cheerful, and always lifts my spirits, especially when I am having a bad day.

What is the difference? Attitude. We will talk more about that later, but your mindset will direct your thoughts. Why is it so hard for some of us to have a good attitude? There are many reasons, but a big one is adverse childhood experiences, or ACE. Any significant stress you go through early in life reshapes your brain to increase your emotional reactivity. Your amygdala, the emotional center of your brain, becomes supercharged. This is one of the things that happens in post-traumatic stress disorder, or PTSD. Small events create a large emotional reaction, often way out of proportion. And this can make you physically sick in addition to psychologically sick.

A study published in 1998 looked at whether stress as a child predicted diseases later in life.[10] It looked for stressors such as abuse (physical, emotional or sexual) or a parent with substance abuse or mental illness. The results were startling. People who had experienced four or more types of ACE were significantly more likely than those without ACE to have heart disease, cancer, chronic chronic lung disease, or liver disease, as well as psychological conditions like alcoholism, drug abuse, or suicide attempts. Childhood stress damages your brain. In medicine, we often see a connection between childhood abuse and depression and anxiety as an adult. Brain neurons have been rewired from the way they are supposed to be. Another well-known paper underscores the importance of a healthy childhood to adult health:

> "Advances in neuroscience, molecular biology, and genomics have converged on three compelling conclusions:
>
> 1. Early experiences are built into our bodies;
>
> 2. Significant adversity can produce physiologic disruptions or biological memories that undermine the development of the body's stress response systems and affect the developing brain, cardiovascular system, immune system, and metabolic regulatory controls;
>
> 3. These physiologic disruptions can persist far into adulthood and lead to lifelong impairments in both physical and mental health."[11]

There are several childhood stressors that impact adult mental and physical health. Certainly, abuse in the household is one of the more problematic ones, in addition to parental mental illness and addiction. However, other common stressors include extreme poverty, community crime, loss of a loved one, frequent relocations, life threatening injuries or diseases, exposure to pornography, peer rejection, and experiencing a natural disaster.

This is a concept that cannot be overemphasized. Stress as a child causes actual brain dysfunction. Mental health issues such as depression, anxiety, or addiction have a very real physical basis. If you had a terrible childhood, does that mean you're stuck? No! We are making real progress in deciphering the brain changes that contribute to mental illness. However, intentional changes in thoughts and behavior are equally important, as any therapist will tell you.

In recent years, we have learned a lot about the tremendous ability of the brain to remodel and heal. You can change your attitude and your thoughts, which will change your brain. We can also use nutritional changes with supplements to heal the brain. It might take a little time and effort, but with God, all things are possible!

More Toxins

We live in a world filled with toxins. One of my colleagues jokes that we are fish and the world is our tank, but no one is cleaning the tank. You usually can't see or smell toxins, but they are there. They are in the air we breathe, both indoors and outdoors. It is widely accepted in the medical field that our water and food supply has been contaminated with toxins. Phthalates, parabens, pesticides, volatile organic compounds, and many more permeate our environment. Our natural environment has changed, and we are suffering for it. These are no longer just intermittent, mild exposures—we are constantly exposed. Those of us who work in integrative medicine see every day what damage toxins can do. We see toxins cause headaches, fatigue, digestive symptoms, thyroid issues, and hormone imbalances.

If you aren't so sure about this crazy "toxin" theory, research what different toxins do. They affect a lot of different things in your body. They can affect the mitochondria in your cells, which are the main "engine" of the cell. This can cause fatigue and muscle soreness. Toxins also can cause gastrointestinal inflammation and a change in the bacteria of your gut, called Dysbiosis.

The result is digestive symptoms and nutrient deficiencies, since you can't absorb nutrients across your intestinal wall as well. You suffer from widespread inflammation, which not only causes aches and pains but also affects brain function. Other toxins directly affect the nervous system, which can cause headaches, numbness, tingling or balance issues.

The more your body is exposed to toxins, the harder it is for your brain to respond to stress. While we have detoxification systems that our cells use to neutralize and eliminate toxins, we are genetically unique. Several genes have common variations that affect the ability to detoxify. If you have a lot of these variations, your body will have a much harder time with the detoxification process.

Some people are genetically susceptible to mold toxins because of the way their immune cells recognize and remove mold toxins. They develop a form of chronic fatigue called Chronic Inflammatory Response Syndrome (CIRS), which is sometimes just called "mold illness" by medical professionals. This can cause different symptoms in different bodies, but most people have severe fatigue, achiness, brain fog and mood changes. We call it a "brain on fire" because the brain has high inflammation and it just doesn't work well. This can also happen after Lyme disease and COVID-19. Inflammation in the brain is not good and affects how you react to stress.

Toxin exposure can fool the best of us. Years ago, we lived in a wonderful home out in the woods in the country. Our back deck looked out on a creek, a small bluff, and the woods. It was just beautiful, but it was built over a natural spring. We started having water issues in that house—first in the crawl space and the basement, then in the bathroom, and then in the garage. We fixed the issues as we found them (or so we thought) but were totally unaware that some mold was still there and was making us sick.

I was tired, but assumed that was because I was raising four children, one with severe autism who usually didn't sleep through the night. I also was working in my solo practice, trying to make enough money to pay the bills. *Talk about high stress!* The other thing that I didn't realize at the time was that I always felt so much better at work. My office was in a small building that we had gutted and renovated, so there was no mold. I would get a lot of energy and my brain would feel just great at work. But then at night, I would crash and get depressed. At church, I used to get so discouraged wondering what was wrong with me. I felt like such a failure for not feeling the joy everyone else was enjoying. Clearly, I was the problem, if everyone else was clapping and shouting for joy in a spirit-filled service, right? Guilt made the depression even worse, but I just didn't know what was wrong.

Now I realize it was being in an environment filled with mold toxins! Back then, I thought I was just weak or simply not good enough. Mold toxins are debilitating to your brain. I had very little stress resilience then. I would snap at my kids or burst into tears when something wasn't working right, and I was deeply depressed much of the time when I was at home. Irritability and depression may be a sign of brain inflammation from mold or other toxins.

If you think you may have mold illness, you can learn more at surviving-mold.com or iseai.org. Most physicians know nothing about mold illness, so you'll have to look carefully for a provider that has had functional training in it. Similarly, if you think you may have chronic Lyme Disease, regular tests done by regular doctors are often falsely negative. Check out ilads.org for resources for testing and treatment.

Other common sources of toxins are exposure to vehicle exhaust, paints or stains, nail or hair salons, frequent use of scented home or beauty products, drinking unfiltered or water bottled in plastics, eating out frequently, use of pesticides in your home, use of herbicides in your landscaping, mercury amalgams in your teeth, or any other chemical occupational exposure. There are also a lot of toxins in our food supply. Glyphosate is in most grains, arsenic contaminates rice, and canned goods can have BPA from the cans leach into the food. I wrote about this in my book *Dare to Detox*. Water and air often have contaminants in them as well. Any of these toxins may be affecting your ability to handle stress.

While we simply cannot eliminate all toxins, we can test for some of them and then work on reducing our exposure. Work with a functional medicine provider to detoxify. If this is affecting you and you don't address it, you will probably continue to feel stressed and won't get the victory you are entitled to.

More Medications

All the reasons we have looked at contribute to stress today. But sometimes we don't realize how bad it is for others, because so many are on medication for anxiety or depression. I go into more detail in Chapter 2, but when I was in primary care, probably about a third of my patients were on medication for anxiety, depression, or sleep. While medications may help, most of the time they are not getting to the root of the problem. They bandage a non-healing wound. Now don't get me wrong, I've written hundreds and probably thousands of prescriptions for these meds, and they were warranted. But now that I practice integrative medicine, I have time with my patients to look for the real underlying reason for their mood changes. I love being able to help people wean off medication. Keep in mind, too, that being on an antidepressant sometimes feeds stress, because you know the underlying issue is still there.

When I first became a Christian and then went to medical school, the prevailing attitudes about mental health issues were very different in the church world. I remember many preachers teaching that you don't need antidepressants; *you just need Jesus!* The clear message was that medication was for spiritual weaklings and we all just needed to pray more, pray harder, and believe God more strongly (and maybe throw in a three-day fast if you're really desperate) and God will heal you! If you did take antidepressants, you obviously weren't as spiritually strong as you should be. This harsh judgmental attitude drove many people out of church.

We have come a long way in the past several decades. It is much more common and socially acceptable to take medication for anxiety or depression. Thankfully, it's been a long time since I've heard a preacher shaming someone for taking them. But we need to understand that medication isn't supposed to be a permanent fix. As a Christian physician, I see clearly how antidepressants should point us toward a larger view that looks for other strategies we can incorporate to heal.

Antidepressants typically do calm down emotional reactivity. Instead of getting anxious, frustrated, or depressed when something goes wrong, you are better able to handle stress. That is often a welcome benefit when you are under high stress. However, they often blunt emotions a lot, numbing the pain. To some degree, we need to feel pain to move forward and fix what is causing the pain. Too often, medication allows you to ignore conflict or behaviors and the need to make effective changes.

Antidepressants also blunt the good emotions. Even though you don't feel the lows as much, the medication blunts the highs as well, so you feel flat overall. You lose the ability to experience fullness of joy that Paul tells us about: "Now may the God of hope fill you with all joy and peace in believing, that you may abound in hope by the power of the Holy Spirit" (Romans 15:13). Antidepressants can prevent you from experiencing the abundance of hope, joy, and peace that God intends for us.

These medications can also cause side effects such as sleep issues, weight gain or sexual difficulties. When you study how many of them work, it becomes clear that they may not be good for your brain long-term. We really don't know how they work, beyond the theory that they keep serotonin (the neurotransmitter that gives you calm well-being) in the synapse (nerve connection space) longer. While this theory hasn't been proven, the concern I have is that whatever they are doing to the neurons is also affecting their function in a way that isn't natural. We know that sometimes it is difficult to wean off these medications, so there can be long-lasting effects.

If you are on antidepressants, continue them as directed by your doctor. If it helps your stress resilience, then it probably is worthwhile for now. I do not recommend changing your medication when you are going through something highly stressful. The right time to do so is when your stress is down and you are feeling good emotionally. But optimal health is when your brain is healthy enough to not need medication.

When you and your doctor feel it is a good time to stop your medication, get your body and brain as toxin-free as possible. I have helped countless people clean up their bodies and diets and get the right nutrients into their system, which enabled them to wean off their psychiatric medications. God designed our body and our brains to work in a way that requires a lot of nutrients: proteins, healthy fats, fiber, antioxidants, vitamins, minerals. If you eat white bread, commercial meat, unhealthy fats, and sugar all day long, it should be less of a surprise when your brain doesn't work quite right. We'll get into nutrition a little later, because it is crucial to improving your ability to manage stress. But if you're drinking a soda or sweet tea right now, throw it out and get a glass of filtered water with lemon. Your brain will thank you.

More Crime, Conflict and Corruption

Crime has skyrocketed in recent years. We have come a long way from the idyllic town of Mayberry! Major cities across the US are now run by politicians who, for political reasons, are soft on crime. They have reduced bail requirements, they don't prosecute crimes, and they even let criminals out of jail. This has been growing for some time, but the riots in 2020 brought it out in the open. Senseless violence under the guise of protest caused widespread destruction in many cities.

Chicago has the sad distinction of being one of the most unsafe cities in the nation. The murder rate in the city is completely unacceptable in a developed nation. Yet criminals run the streets, and the police seem to be wholly unable to restrain them. Homelessness has taken over many cities. In particular, Los Angeles and San Francisco are overrun with homeless people on the sidewalks. It's shocking that hard-working Americans have to step over needles and walk around individuals living on the sidewalks right in front of their businesses. Entire sections of cities have been filled with homeless encampments and are now no longer pleasant places to live and raise a family. Sadly, real solutions seem to evade these city leaders.

Even worse, we as citizens have been awakened to a seditious amount of corruption within the media, the government, the banking industry, politicians, and many major corporations. This adds to our stress, as we see clearly that there are indeed many evil people in this world, and their only goal is power and control. We are expendable in their minds, and their decisions affect our daily lives in very difficult and painful ways.

We are warned that, in the last days, "Evil men and seducers shall wax worse and worse, deceiving, and being deceived" (2 Tim 3:13 KJV). There has been evil in this world for millennia, but it's more pervasive now, and we are exposed to so much more of it. With technology and instant news reporting, we see reports of evil constantly. We can see stories of evil from across the world on social media on our phones. Images and stories of corruption and violence can easily fill our minds if we let them in. Most of us have had to teach our children how to limit media and exposure to certain things. When I was young, that meant not seeing an R-rated movie until I was well into high school. Now it's a Herculean task monitoring our children's cell phones and social media. It is just so easy for them to see things that are not good for their development or their souls. We must discipline ourselves, too. Turn off your cell phone and unplug from social media and all the negativity on the news occasionally. If all you put in your heart is bad news, how can you possibly expect to feel peace and joy? Stop adding to your stress with what you watch on television or online. Look to Jesus, the One who gives us hope, no matter what is going on around us.

More Acceptable So We Recognize It Less

We can see stress is so common that we don't appreciate how much of a problem it is. We simply accept it as normal. I am completely guilty of this. As an overachiever, I think my brain has been programmed to push through adversity, no matter how tough the situation, and to just deal with discomfort. I studied for hours in high school and got straight A's. I worked hard in college to get the grades I needed to go to medical school. Then in med school, wow! You had to study every night until late at night just to keep up with the new material that had been presented that day. Clinical rotations were worse: working thirty-six-hour shifts as a student wasn't much fun. Then residency was even harder: thirty-six-hour shifts every three days as an intern for a whole year. Sleep was a rare treat, and you just had no choice but to push on and do what had to be done.

But if you had asked any of us if we were stressed, we would just laugh. Of course we were stressed! But what choice did we have? Many of us would answer the question the same: We bear heavy loads but just accept it as a normal part of life. Many of us just don't realize the magnitude of our stress. When we are blinded to our stress and our reactions, we move through life on autopilot. We react according to our emotions and just try to get through. This causes poor brain health and worsening coping skills. Before we realize it, we are in a deep pit, and we don't even look up to see the trees and the sky above our head. We run around in circles, knowing we aren't living a joy-filled victorious life, but not sure why or what to do. We must first do a lot of honest self-evaluation to really assess how we are doing.

I have a friend who has gone to Costa Rica a few times on yoga retreats. She doesn't watch television; she spends hours relaxing and is almost completely unplugged from the world. Compare that life to my typical days and wow, my stress is pretty obvious!

I would encourage you to take a day or a weekend to really spend some time alone and think about this. Go for a walk, take a bath, or take a friend out for coffee. Examine all the areas of your life that are stressful, whether it inherently is or if it's something you make worse. So first, honestly assess what your stressors are. *Spouse? Boss? Job responsibilities or co-workers? Church mismanagement? Annoying mother-in-law?* Write them all down— all of them you can possibly think of.

You might be surprised how much you write down, because we tend to deny how much things stress us. Once you have listed them all, take out a highlighter and highlight the ones you have no control over. For example, a lazy co-worker who doesn't pull their weight, the winter weather if you live in Minnesota, or a loved one with a chronic illness. Then, for all the ones left, think about two things:

> » Is there anything I can do that will possibly make the situation better?

> » If I can't change the situation at all, how am I responding to it? How can I react better?

For example, having an infant is just stressful because of the demands. It is what it is. But if you have a sixteen-year-old with ADHD who won't do his homework, and you feel like you must nag him and sit with him every night to get his homework done, realize that you are choosing to make your evenings stressful. There are other ways to deal with problem behavior that don't emotionally drain you, especially with a teenager.

My husband and I are raising a child with autism. Anyone who has a child with special needs, whether physical or developmental, knows all too well how challenging it can be. I remember, when our son Daniel was young and never slept through the night, thinking that it would have been amazing to have a "normal" baby who only disrupted our sleep until around six months old. That would have been nothing compared to all the years we spent with him waking up at night. Add to that behavioral and school challenges, and any special needs parent becomes a superhero of sorts. We do it because we love our child, but often we also underestimate how stressed we are.

I have a friend whose middle schooler frequently forgot her lunch or schoolwork and would then call to ask her mom bring it to her. One year, she decided to tell her daughter on the first day of school, "I will bring something to you once and only once as an act of grace. Anything forgotten after that will have consequences, and you are responsible for those." It only took until the second week of school for her to hit that wall. When she forgot something, she was astounded her mom held firm, despite her insistence about how she would get points marked off. It was hard for mom, but guess what? It worked beautifully! It only took a few times for her daughter to realize that she and she alone had to be responsible.

What are you doing for your kids that they should do? Laundry, dishes, or cleaning? My kids started doing their own laundry at age five. I had enough to do, and they were quite capable of washing and drying their clothes. They learned to help with meal prep in the kitchen, they always helped with dishes, and they had to pick up their things every night. I'm not saying they were great at their chores or that they always had a good attitude, but I sure wasn't going to do all the work after being in my office for ten hours. I learned early on that I needed to come home and relax if I was going to be any good to anyone else the next day.

Another situation that required adjustment was when my dad's heart failure was getting worse the last few years of his life. He and his doctors had a lot of trouble keeping fluid out of his lungs while keeping his kidneys working. His anxiety got worse the last few years, essentially because he knew he was dying, and he was not ready for that. He would call me and ask me a lot of detailed questions about his lab values and medications. This created high stress for me, because I wasn't his doctor and couldn't answer most of his questions.

I couldn't change what was happening to him. I tried my best to answer his questions, but I realized one day that he really didn't want to know why his creatinine level went up. He was just anxious about dying and focused on the details of his medical condition as a coping mechanism. Like a child hearing thunder in the middle of the night, he wanted to be told it was all going to be okay. I started deflecting his questions from the specifics into reassuring generalities, and it seemed to help his high anxiety come down. We couldn't change his condition, but we both could change our thoughts and our speech. We started to talk about dying and faith, and that was so much more needful than me answering medical questions.

I changed my approach with Dad to try to not enable his anxiety, but to bring him peace. He was anxious and dying slowly, and my mom was taking care of him around the clock, so that situation wasn't changeable. But I had to take special time to care for myself spiritually and mentally before and after interacting with Mom or Dad. *You can change how you react.* We all grieved when Dad passed away, but we chose to celebrate a life well-lived.

Stress can shape you, grow you, and help you become who you are supposed to be. It's all in your reaction to it. When you are honest with yourself, you will see how you can handle stress better. Sometimes you need to say no to further commitments. Sometimes it's going to bed earlier with a good book. Sometimes it's choosing to overlook a hurtful comment. Sometimes it's fully forgiving someone of deep hurt.

Your first step in overcoming is recognizing truly what your stress is. The second is realizing how you are reacting to it. You will not overcome and grow into what God has planned for you until you are honest with yourself and God.

CHAPTER 2

How Stress Is Killing Us

Before we talk more about how to deal with stress, we need to take a hard look at what stress does to us. Most people know that stress causes anxiety, depression, headaches, and ulcers, but it goes far beyond that. Stress can affect every organ system in your body. I'm probably going to scare you a little bit to help motivate you to take this seriously. Once you understand how much stress can do, I'll give you a road map that will guide you to a place of physical, mental, and spiritual health.

Mental Health

Stress is widely believed to be the biggest medical challenge of our day. We have antibiotics, open-heart surgery, and clot-dissolving medications that save lives every day. But stress is a leading cause of mood disorders and cognitive decline. Our brains are suffering.

We are seeing an epidemic of depression and anxiety. When I was in medical school, Prozac® had recently come on to the market. Until then, we only had the older antidepressants that were not very good. You had to push the doses up high to get relief of depression, and most people got constipation, sedation, or even trouble urinating. Quite often, the medication wasn't worth the side effects. But then Prozac® became available, and it seemed to make a significant difference in mood without all of the adverse side effects.

Fast forward several decades, and it seems that a whole lot of people have been on some psychiatric medication at one time or another.

A study done in 2013 showed that 16.7 percent of adults filled at least one prescription for a psychiatric drug that year.[12] 12 percent were for antidepressants, 8 percent were for anxiety medications or sedatives, and 1.6 percent were for antipsychotics. I often think about (*here we go again!*) our response to what's going on in our mind. Do we look for any pill we can get? What about exercise? Changing nutrition? Seeing a therapist? You may have brain inflammation causing mood changes from something that you had no control over, but you can change how you handle it. The stark reality is that a majority of us have had symptoms of a mental health disorder at some point. It's an epidemic!

What does stress do to the brain? Studies have shown that repeated patterns of thought create entrenched pathways in the brain that are very hard to change. For example, if your father was physically abusive, and every time he came home angry, he slammed his keys down on the counter, how would you react? You would learn quickly what the sound of the keys meant and you would tense up. Your heart rate and breathing would accelerate. Your body would pump out adrenaline to increase your alertness for danger. Cortisol would also be released, which would prevent you from relaxing for hours afterward. For the rest of your life, when someone lays their keys down hard, you may jump and get a similar physical reaction. That response in brain pathways is entrenched to warn you about impending danger. This may lessen over time, but sometimes it never fully goes away. This is what happens in PTSD. A trigger like the original stressor triggers the same physical and emotional reaction. Soldiers often cannot handle thunderstorms or fireworks. It's just too much like what they experienced in combat. A fun summer picnic in July triggers a rush of adrenaline and cortisol that washes over the brain, hijacking normal, rational thought. In my case, my son with autism also has seizures. The first few he had were so bad that he had to be rushed to the hospital, where they put him under deep sedation and on a respirator to control the seizures. Those were bad. Now his seizures are different: they don't last long, and then he sleeps it off. But when he makes a weird sound or I hear a loud noise from his room, I immediately rush in to make sure he's not having a seizure. My brain is just wired to be constantly on alert for sounds that might indicate a problem.

It doesn't take severe stress to rewire your brain. Even small stresses, over time, can change your thoughts if you're not careful. As stress continues, it is easy to lose hope that things will ever get better. This is a leading cause of depression. Never forget that your emotions are tightly related to your thoughts, which can be either bad or good. Psychologists make a living by helping you purposefully change your thoughts. Negative thoughts lead to negative emotions. Not feeling grounded and confident leads to anxiety. Poor self-esteem and not knowing who you are in God's kingdom leads to anxiety. Chronic anxiety leads to depression.

Remember the example of the teenager with ADD that you think you have to help with his homework every night? You incorrectly assume responsibility (wrong thought), which makes you feel guilty if you don't act on it (negative emotion). This causes stress (you don't want to do it but feel obligated, and then you are exhausted and feel taken advantage of). This neural pattern of wrong thoughts causing negative emotions becomes entrenched. But if someone says "What on earth are you doing? Quit it and let him fail if he doesn't do it!"—you may be stunned but intrigued. Do it, and you will be pleasantly surprised to find that your stress is much better. You may not even need your antidepressant or your sleeping pill. And even better, you'll feel empowered and more in control of your life.

Beyond mood disorders, stress causes inflammation in the brain that affects memory, focus and cognitive processing. Have you ever had test anxiety? This is the classic example of how mental stress can make it harder for you to think quickly, logically, and correctly. I have taken more tests in my lifetime than most and still take exams from time to time to maintain my certifications. In the old days, you would have about six or seven hours of testing in a day, with breaks, and it was usually plenty of time. Now, testing is often done online sitting at a computer with a timer. One test I recently took allowed five minutes per question. For some questions, it was not at all a problem. But for some of the complex ones with a lot of data to review and sort through, I got panicky after three minutes. (For math folks, one was a very tricky statistics question about specificity, sensitivity, positive predictive value, and negative predictive value. My brain hurt.) By the time the screen was flashing and counting down from fifty-nine seconds to zero, I could tell my brain wasn't really weighing all the details very rationally. I ended up just picking an answer because my brain couldn't think clearly with the timer flashing down!

Imagine feeling a bit of that stress all the time. It is not good for your brain. You may or may not notice an effect, but every day I have patients tell me their memory isn't as good as it used to be, or they have trouble staying on task, or they just don't feel like their brain is as sharp as it should be. We'll talk about this later in the chapter, but stress shrinks the cells of the hippocampus, which is the part of the brain that creates and retrieves memory. We think it is because, when there is inflammation in the brain, the brain cells actually shrink to protect themselves from the inflamma-tion. It is a preservation response, but after a while, the total volume of the hippocampus decreases and your memory suffers. The other effect of shrinkage in the hippocampus is that you have less cells in your memory center to interpret your environment and judge whether something is a stressor. This can increase the stress response, which creates a vicious cycle, making it even worse! Overall, your brain just doesn't work optimally when you're stressed. You can weather this for a short time, but long term, it increases your risk for dementia. There is a lot of research going on now in Alzheimer's disease. The biochemistry is fascinating to see, especially the link between inflammation and changes seen in Alzheimer's. We know stress leads to inflammation, so it just isn't good for brain function.

Physical Health

Estimates for primary care say about 60-80 percent of what a typical primary care physician sees in any day is either caused or affected by stress.[13] I believe this! I practiced as a family physician for twenty years. About

10-20 percent of the diagnoses I dealt with every day included depression, anxiety, or insomnia. But if you look deeper, many other conditions are affected by stress.

Stress affects your immune system, your brain function, and your hormones, and it contributes to inflammation, which can destroy your body. I would venture to say that most disease we see, while not necessarily caused by stress, is affected by stress. And that's a direct medical/biological effect on the disease process. I'm not even talking about the psychological effect of having a chronic disease and how that causes stress and is worsened by having a high stress load. Most family physicians will tell you that if stress was wiped out and people ate healthy, whole food diets, they would probably go out of business. That's how powerful diet and stress management are.

One of my favorite scriptures is this: "It is the glory of God to conceal a matter, but the glory of kings is to search out a matter" (Proverbs 25:2). God designed our bodies and minds to work in a certain way, and we need to dig deep to figure out what is happening when we are stressed and what to do about it. Let's get started.

Sleep

Sleep is a precious thing! We all know what it's like to fall into bed after a long day filled with fun, social connections and physical activity. For example, if you have a big picnic with your family, filled with swimming and water skiing, you'll probably sleep well that night. You will wake up eight to nine hours later feeling refreshed and ready for a new day. That's what God intended. He didn't design us to stay up until midnight on our computers or watching television, blue light hitting our eyeballs, then toss and turn all night with stressful thoughts, only to wake up at six in the morning to be at work by seven.

Matthew Walker, PhD wrote a book called *Why We Sleep*. It is a deep dive into what happens in our brain when we sleep. It includes a lot of the science of sleep, which we biology geeks find fascinating.[14] He explains the different phases of sleep (REM and NREM) and what happens during each phase. He makes a very compelling case for how crucial it is that we get a full, deep, restful night's sleep every night for our brains to work normally. Dr. Walker talks about research that shows even one night of disrupted sleep lowers brain function for days afterward. He shows why you just can't skimp on sleep during the week and expect to catch up on the weekends—it has been proven not to work.

Dr. Walker explains how your brain is weakened without good sleep. You don't think clearly, you have poorer logical skills, and your focus is just terrible when you don't sleep. It's like you have early dementia! How on earth do you think you'll be able to give a coherent, vibrant presentation when you didn't sleep enough? How will you handle an irritable toddler when you are irritable yourself? I can't emphasize enough how crucial it is that you sleep well.

When I see patients complaining of fatigue, brain fog, or weight gain, I always address sleep right away. I recently saw a new patient, a fifty-five-year-old woman whose main complaints were afternoon fatigue, difficulty losing weight, and poor sleep. After getting a complete history and getting her set up for comprehensive testing, she casually mentioned that she had been diagnosed with sleep apnea. She had a CPAP machine but didn't like it, so she stopped using it. Because she shared this detail at the end of her appointment, I took a little more time to tell her that, if she had apnea (which causes low oxygen to the brain all night long), she would not feel better as long as she refused to treat it. She would continue to be tired and overweight, and no prescription pill would fix it.

There is no magic hormone that will give you energy, sharpen your brain, and make you lose weight if you are not sleeping well. It's like thinking that Diet Coke makes up for the cookies you eat every day. It doesn't work! If you want more energy and a healthy brain, you must sleep at least six hours of sleep, but eight is better.

A lot of people come to me with difficulty losing weight, and they hope bioidentical hormone therapy will cause weight loss. While balanced hormones are essential, a common reason for the inability to lose weight is poor sleep. I have seen a lot of people eating a very healthy, low-carb, reduced calorie diet but they will not lose weight if they aren't sleeping well. It turns out that poor sleep is associated with decreased leptin.

Leptin and ghrelin are two hormones involved with hunger and fat burning or storage. Leptin makes you feel full and allows your body to burn your fat for fuel. Leptin is produced at night during deep sleep. Ghrelin is the opposite. It causes you to feel hungry, and your body thinks it's time to eat. When you eat, the extra energy is then stored, but you really didn't need it. When your sleep is disrupted, leptin goes down and ghrelin goes up. That's why you get hungry at one in the morning when you can't sleep and why you can't lose weight.

The scary thing is that lack of sleep is strongly correlated with heart disease,[15] stroke,[16] diabetes,[17] dementia,[18] and obesity.[19] Not getting enough sleep can cause inflammation, which disrupts many of the body's normal processes, increasing pain in muscles or joints, causing headaches, or even digestive symptoms.

Should you just take a sleeping pill, if sleep is that important? No. They aren't good for you. Natural sleep is so healing and so restorative, and sleep induced by a drug is not the same. Sleeping pills change the way you sleep, and you do not get the same restorative effect. In fact, benzodiazepines, such as alprazolam, increase your risk for dementia. *Yikes!* You thought not sleeping made you crazy; well, taking meds isn't much better in the long run. If you are currently taking something for sleep, discuss it with your doctor. I usually tell my new patients that if they are working, it's okay to continue them while you work on all the other things you can do. The ultimate goal is to replace them with natural supplements or even to get off them totally, but it is a process, so just keep the goal in mind. We will talk about some natural options a bit later.

Fatigue

Beyond poor sleep, everyone seems tired these days. Almost all my new patients report low energy levels. We all hate being tired, because we remember what it's like to have a lot of energy and feel full of life. Remember long summer days when you were a kid? I could spend the whole morning outside running around playing. We'd come in for lunch and supper, but otherwise we would be outside all day. We had lots of energy! *Those were the days, right?* So many things drain our energy. Poor nutrition, poor sleep and inflammation, but stress is a big cause.

It starts as mental fatigue. You are so frustrated at what is not right in life that you lose motivation and mental energy. It's easier to sit and watch television. It takes too much energy to socialize or do something productive. Over time, when your mental energy is low, your physical energy drops, and you just can't get off the couch. You may come home from work and crash after dinner. Remember when you were a young adult and would go out with your friends at nine at night? I can hear you parents laughing now. That's pajama time for many of you!

Fatigue can be a good thing, but often it is not God's will. If you worked hard all day, fatigue is the normal response for you to rest so your body can rejuvenate. But if it happens for no reason day after day, I will say it is not God's plan for your life. God wants us energized and able to minister and do His work every day. How are you going to notice that a friend is a little down and needs encouragement if you're exhausted? How are you going to be used to bless others if you're focused on how tired you are? God's ultimate plan is that He works through us. We are His hands and feet, and His Spirit works through us in connection with others. But we need to be healthy and have enough energy to be useful to Him.

God wants us to trust Him so we can have His peace. He is the Prince of Peace, Jehovah Shalom. That name is one of my favorite names for God. Although sin has entered the world and now we are surrounded by toxins, nutrient depleted food, and stress, God has made a way for our brains and emotions to work well. You don't have to suffer from depression or anxiety. God's will is for you to be healthy in all ways. "Beloved, I pray that you may prosper in all things and be in health, just as your soul prospers" (3 John 1:2).

Cortisol and Hormones

When you are stressed, your hormones will be affected. That's a certainty. The first system that is affected is cortisol, but that can affect your sex hormones and then your thyroid, so the result is a mess.

Your adrenal glands make a hormone called cortisol. Cortisol is a natural part of how we respond to stress. It isn't bad at all; it is a useful hormone.

We just need certain amounts of it and stress often makes it too high or too low. The adrenal glands also make adrenaline (or epinephrine), which is part of the fight or flight system, but the effects of adrenaline should be short lived. Adrenaline is released in microseconds in response to a threat. This is what causes your heart rate to skyrocket, bringing an immediate sense of alarm. It should subside quickly after the threat goes away. Cortisol is a stress hormone released more slowly in response to a threat, and it takes much longer to subside, which can cause problems if the stress is persistent.

Chronic stress affects cortisol through a system called the hypothalamic-pituitary-adrenal axis, or "HPA axis." Here's how it works:

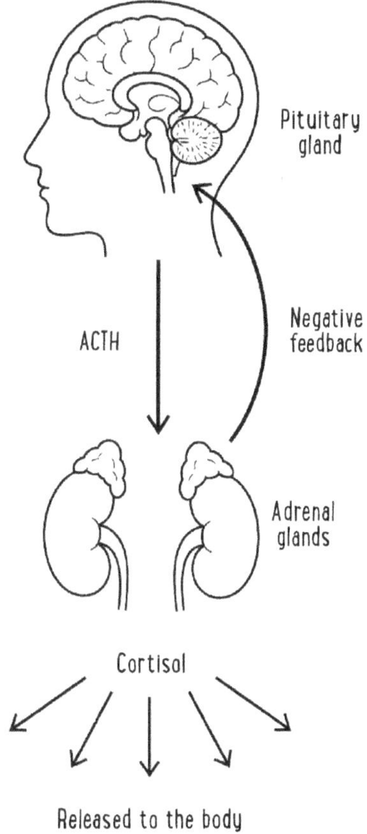

HYPOTHALAMIC-PITUITARY-ADRENAL AXIS

Cortisol then goes throughout your body to do three things:

1. Increases adrenaline
2. Increases blood sugar
3. Decreases inflammation

Cortisol plays a vital role in helping you cope with a stressful situation. It increases alertness, gets your muscles tensed and ready for action, increases your blood sugar level so your cells have fuel, and increases your heart rate and blood pressure so you will have the blood circulation to do what you have to do. However, once the stress has subsided, cortisol should go down to normal. The way this happens is that when cortisol levels are high, they act on the brain to suppress further production of ACTH and thus, less cortisol is made.

For example, when you work out, your body will produce a surge of cortisol. This is a normal response. But within several hours after your workout, your cortisol should drop back down to a normal level. This also should happen if something happens that is bad. Let's say you have a minor car accident. When it first happens, your adrenaline levels spike within seconds. That will subside within a few hours. But cortisol will be strongly released in the first few hours and often will stay high for a day or two, even after you feel like you have calmed down. But if the stress subsides, your cortisol levels will also decrease. Now let's say you have a very stressful job. Your cortisol will be high all day long and even into the evening, which will prevent you from relaxing and sleeping well. Your cortisol may even stay high on the weekend. It could take a week of vacation for them to become normal.

Early in the stress response, cortisol levels tend to be high. But over time, your levels tend to drop low. We used to call this "adrenal fatigue." Then we realized that people with high cortisol often have similar symptoms to people with low cortisol. High cortisol does often cause the "wired but tired" feeling with irritability, frustration, and anxiety. But most of those people also say they are tired.

Low cortisol levels are typically seen with chronic stress. When cortisol is low throughout the day, most people feel chronically fatigued. They can be depressed and have significant brain fog. Most of us no longer call this "adrenal fatigue" but instead use the term "HPA axis dysfunction," which is short for hypothalamic-pituitary-adrenal axis dysfunction. It is more descriptive of the fact that it's not just that cortisol is high or low, but it's the whole system that is off somehow. Another term sometimes used is "hypocortisolism," describing when cortisol is chronically low.

Our thinking about adrenals has evolved in recent years. We now realize that we have been blaming the adrenal glands for years, but the new name highlights that the problem really is starting in the brain. Even through stress, the adrenals could and do make cortisol with the right signal. But the brain isn't doing its job correctly.

Here's a key fact: brain inflammation is often the root of cortisol issues. When your brain is inflamed, the hypothalamus and pituitary do not send the proper signal to the adrenals. It's like when the parents leave teenagers at home alone. They will come home to a house with dirty dishes, warm milk on the counter, and dishes in the living room. There was no direction from the parents to tell them to do what they were supposed to do. When your brain is on fire from inflammation, it affects your cortisol levels. The brain just doesn't send the right signal to the adrenals to make proper amounts of cortisol.

When you get your cortisol checked, it may tell you several things:

1. Something is not normal

2. Cortisol is overall trending high or trending low

3. Your cortisol curve is flat

We will talk about ways to test your cortisol a little later. But I'll tell you now, it's not just about testing one level. We want to see how your cortisol levels are through the day, because they are supposed to rise within two hours of waking up and then slowly decrease through the day until bedtime. Variations in this "cortisol curve" are often quite telling and help us pinpoint where in the day stress is affecting you the most.

Sex Hormones

The next type of hormone affected by stress is sex hormones. These include estrogen, testosterone, progesterone, and DHEA for both men and women. When your hypothalamus and pituitary gland are affected by stress, they are "downregulated," meaning they do not send enough signal to the ovaries or testes, so hormone production goes down.

For example, when cortisol is high, it tells the pituitary to make less ACTH. This can cause the pituitary to make less LH and FSH (pituitary hormones), which then results in less estrogen and testosterone production. For example, when women have high stress, they often will not have the right amount of LH and FSH made, so they don't ovulate. This causes irregular periods and can affect fertility. In men, testosterone levels can drop.

When women don't have enough estrogen, they can have hot flashes, night sweats, insomnia, and brain fog. When their progesterone levels fall, mood swings and sleep trouble are common. When testosterone levels fall in either men or women, libido drops and sexual health suffers.

There is another way stress can affect your hormones. Sometimes, I put people on bioidentical hormones, and I can get their levels well into the normal range, but they don't feel any better. This happens a lot with testosterone. People under stress sometimes need higher doses of testosterone to help them with their low sex drive, low motivation and brain fog. Why is that? We think it is because stress affects the way testosterone works on the cellular level. The testosterone must get into the cell and then go to the nucleus, where it interacts with DNA to eventually cause a protein to be made which has an effect. There are a lot of things that can break down in this chain of events. When you are inflamed or stressed, this process can be affected. Clinically, we see that regular doses of testosterone sometimes just don't work as well. We need to use higher doses to see an effect. And then we sometimes deal with side effects. If you are stressed and have poor lifestyle habits, please don't ask for your "magic testosterone" prescription. It is much more effective to work on stress reduction and stress management, together with sleep and nutrition, first.

Sometimes, hormones will improve on their own after those changes. But then if we still have to use hormone therapy, it simply works better.

The other hormonal issue that can be related to stress is infertility. Women need to have regular menstrual cycles with normal ovulation in order to conceive. Stress can alter your estrogen and progesterone, causing a decrease in ovulation and sometimes insufficient hormone levels to support a healthy pregnancy. It is a common finding that, when couples who are struggling with infertility finally stop treatment, they sometimes conceive on their own. The stress goes down, and then it happens!

Thyroid

The next hormone that is affected by stress is the thyroid gland. Your thyroid gland also responds to a pituitary signal, which is called thyroid stimulating hormone, or TSH. You may have had a TSH blood test to check your thyroid. Did you know that TSH is not a thyroid hormone level? It does give us a good idea of your thyroid function, though. TSH tells the thyroid gland to make thyroid hormone, most of which is T4 and T3. T4 is the major one made, and as it travels throughout the body, it is converted to T3, which is the main form that goes into cells to drive cellular energy production.

When you are stressed, cortisol can suppress the pituitary gland overall, resulting in less hormones being made. But stress also affects the crucial conversion of T4 to T3. T4 can be turned into two forms of T3: regular T3 and reverse T3. Reverse T3 is like a mirror image to regular T3. It has the same molecular structure but it's backwards. It is what I call a "dud" form of T3. It doesn't do anything! It will not work in the cells. When you are stressed, more of your T4 becomes reverse T3, so there is less regular, active T3 for your cells. You can also get a type of thyroid receptor resistance. This is hard to diagnose, but sometimes all your thyroid hormone blood levels look fine, but you still have symptoms of low thyroid such as fatigue, weight gain, and constipation. Stress can do that.

Blood Sugar

The last hormonal system affected by stress is blood sugar metabolism. This is the interaction between glucose and insulin. When you eat carbohydrates, whether it is bread or a cookie, it ends up as glucose. Glucose in your blood triggers your pancreas to release insulin. Insulin's job is to go out into the blood and grab on to glucose and pull it into the cells. That's okay if it's going into a brain cell or a muscle cell, but if you just had a combo meal at your favorite drive-through, you may have eaten 200 grams of carbs which is about ten times more than you really needed. All that extra glucose is pulled into the fat cells by insulin. Insulin causes weight gain, which makes you stressed, which makes you miserable, and the cycle repeats. The first step is to reduce carb consumption.

Something else is happening a lot, too: insulin resistance. Nutrient depletion and some toxins cause our insulin to be ineffective. If two people eat the same size serving of rice, one person's blood sugar will go higher, because their insulin doesn't work as well. Their body makes more insulin to compensate for its inefficiency. Elevated insulin sends a powerful signal to the fat cells to hold on to fat and not burn it. Then you can't lose weight or even gain weight.

What does stress have to do with insulin? Remember, cortisol is preparing the body to deal with stress. It thinks you need more glucose in your blood, so it does two things. Firstly, it tells your liver to make and release glucose into the blood. Secondly, it makes fat and muscle cells insulin resistant. Then insulin won't pull glucose in those cells, leaving more in the blood. You have both more glucose in your bloodstream and more insulin, which isn't working very well. Both glucose and insulin are damaging to cells, proteins in particular. Glucose can change the structure of a protein, by a process called "glycation", damaging it permanently. Obesity and inflammation commonly occur from insulin resistance. Combined with a high carbohydrate diet, stress can make you prediabetic. It can even cause diabetes in those who are otherwise predisposed.

Those of us in integrative medicine often refer to the "Adrenal-Thyroid-Pancreas" system, or "stress-metabolism-sugar." These three hormone-producing glands very commonly affect each other. For example, stress happens first. This will raise your blood sugar and drop your thyroid hormone levels. They are all connected.

Brain Changes From Stress

Your brain is affected by stress in ways we are just beginning to understand. We know stress affects neurotransmitters like serotonin and dopamine. To be overly simplistic, when you have low serotonin, you are more likely to be depressed, and when your dopamine is low, you won't feel like doing anything, and you have little joy. But the neurotransmitters are much more complex than that, and stress affects a lot more than neurotransmitters.

We've talked about how stress and negative thoughts change your brain. Remember those adverse childhood experiences, or ACEs we talked about? They rewire your brain. People who suffered trauma or abuse when young often need therapy to help change the pattern of neural connections to healthier thought processes. This can be very powerful. I have patients who have escaped abusive relationships. What do they have in common? They have been intentional in taking care of themselves and healing their emotions and thoughts. They have overcome the bad with good.

On a cellular level, chronic stress causes inflammation in the brain. There are cells called microglial cells, which are immune cells that create inflammation. Stress can be a factor in activating microglial cells. This can cause neural excitability, leading to irritability and mood swings.

On a larger level, chronic stress will shrink the hippocampus, which is the memory center of the brain. It also enlarges the amygdala, which is the part of the brain that monitors for danger. When the amygdala enlarges, it gets overactive. Minor threats are interpreted as severe. You are more edgy and it is more difficult to relax.

One severe form of stress induced dysfunction is PTSD. A lot of people who have had chronic stress combined with a lack of control over their environment have some degree of PTSD. In terms of brain effects, PTSD causes the amygdala to become overreactive. Small, innocuous things create a disproportionate emotional response. But you don't have to have PTSD to have this happen. You can just be having a bad day.

For example, the other day, I had just had it. My son Daniel, who has autism, was displaying a lot of behaviors indicating he just needed constant attention. I had worked all day, cooked dinner, did the dishes, put the clean laundry away, and had just gotten him a snack. I was just about to get a snack for myself and finally sit on the couch and relax, then he came in and signed "drink" (he's mostly nonverbal and uses some signs and his iPad to communicate). I am not proud of myself at all for the way I reacted. But I was already so frazzled and emotionally spent that, before I could think, I said to him, "Dude, you're killing me!" I got up as grumpy as could be and got him his drink of water.

Hard to admit, but my inner child emotions came out under the stress. But only for a moment! I was immediately convicted of my attitude and my frustration. He just wanted water. He didn't understand that I had done too much that day and needed to relax and unwind. He sure didn't deserve my inexcusable reaction. (Fortunately, he didn't notice or care.) I also immediately felt horrible for speaking such negative words. There is a very powerful spiritual principle of speaking life and not negative words. But I realized that there was a nugget of truth in my outburst. Stress can indeed be killing us. Are you letting it kill you?

Immune System

Stress can affect your immune system in many ways. We know that when we are run down, we get colds and viruses more easily. The main reason for this is that, when your cortisol is high, your immune system is suppressed. Cortisone shots into joints and cortisone creams for rashes are anti-inflammatory. When your body makes cortisol, it has the same effect. It suppresses your immune cells so they are less able to fight off infections. Remember the 1980s and 1990s, when we were grappling with the rise in Acquired Immune Deficiency Syndrome, or AIDS? Those of us in medicine then remember it well. This was in the days before we had good medication to treat it. Immune cell counts plummeted, and these people got scary infections and died frequently. In those days, "PCP" meant pneumocystis carinii pneumonia, not primary care physician. We did our best, but a severely weakened immune system often meant death.

Another severe case of immune disease was "Bubble Boy." This was a child with Severe Combined Immune Deficiency, or SCID. He was born in 1971 with SCID, which causes an overall inability to fight off any germ. A simple cold virus would have killed him. He was put in a germ-free bubble at Texas Children's Hospital in Houston. The only treatment available at the time was a bone marrow transplant, but there was no suitable donor. He lived until age twelve when he died of lymphoma.

The other thing that can happen with high cortisol from stress is poor wound healing. When you have an injury or wound, your body creates a massive response of inflammation for a very good reason: the inflammatory cytokines go to work to repair the cells that were damaged. Open blood vessels clot and stop bleeding, white blood cells deal with foreign material and germs, and then new cells can grow and repair the tissue. But if this response is weak, your wound will not heal well. Stress can make you sick and suppress your ability to heal.

Another interesting example is COVID-19. Those who were the most fearful and stressed in the early days of the pandemic often had high cortisol due to their perceived level of stress. High cortisol suppresses the body's ability to fight off infection. Several studies done in 2020 showed significantly higher cortisol levels in those who died compared to those who survived.[20] While the cortisol could have been higher due to being sicker, having high cortisol is known to be immunosuppressive.

On the flip side, researchers are looking at chronically low cortisol being associated with long COVID. This makes sense, because low cortisol often causes fatigue. Low cortisol also causes a weakened immune system, and one theory of long COVID is that it has to do with reactivation of latent viruses such as Epstein-Barr virus. Whether your cortisol is high or low, your immune system may very well be affected in some way.

Disease

There are many diseases that happen from stress. We have talked about hormone issues, sleep, and brain changes. But stress can also make your body susceptible to deadly diseases.

Cancer

Stress can affect the immune issue in a way that leads to cancer. You need certain immune cells and cytokines (inflammatory mediators) to kill off cells when they start to turn cancerous. There is a theory that all of us develop cancer several times in our lifetime. But our immune cells detect those early cancer cells, kill them, and clean up the mess, all unknown to us. But if your immune system is impaired, a few cells could take root and grow.

A study on cortisol patterns found that women with metastatic breast cancer had flattened cortisol curves compared to healthy women.[21] Another study showed that among breast cancer patients, having a flat cortisol curve predicted mortality.[22] One way this can happen is that having a flat cortisol curve is associated with less natural killer (NK) cell activity. NK cells are the good guys, eating up cancer cells. If you don't have NK cells, cancers grow quickly. Stress can reduce NK cell activity, thereby increasing your risk for cancer.

The evidence that chronic stress causes cancer is not completely definitive. There have been studies showing a connection but also some that do not show any connection. This is because cancer is very complex and there are a lot of factors other than stress. I personally believe that, even if you have high stress, the way you react to it can affect whether it will affect your immune system, thus changing your cancer risk. So once again, you might not be able to control the stress, but you can control your reaction to it.

I don't know about you, but I sure don't want to take any chances with increasing my cancer risk. I want my immune system as healthy as it can be. Keep in mind that stress sometimes causes people to smoke, drink alcohol, or eat sugary foods. These behaviors can increase your risk for cancer due to their destructive effects.

If you do have cancer, stress will increase glucose. Sugar feeds cancer. The current thinking in oncology is that a ketogenic diet may be a helpful addition to cancer therapies, because it deprives cancer cells of glucose.[23] When you have cancer and either eat sugar or your cortisol makes sugar, you are feeding your cancer.

Dementia

Dementia can be caused by blood vessel damage and mini-strokes over time, or more commonly by Alzheimer's. This is a complex process where the brain's neurons are progressively damaged. We now know that insulin resistance is linked to dementia. Some doctors even call it "type 3 diabetes," referring to the fact that research has shown that Alzheimer's dementia is from insulin resistance in the brain. If you are stressed a lot and have chronically-elevated cortisol, your insulin resistance affects your whole body, including your brain.

We do see memory issues in people who have chronically high cortisol levels. It is just harder for people to learn new information and recall it. So high cortisol over a long time can't be good for your brain down the road.

But does chronic stress cause dementia? We don't know for sure. Some studies have shown an increased incidence of dementia related to stress. But these types of studies are hard to interpret, because types of stress and people's resilience to stress vary widely. We know some degree of stress is good for your brain. For example, if you retire at age sixty-five and sit in your recliner watching television all day, your brain will atrophy. But if you take up a hobby, learn a new skill, and keep a busy schedule, that small amount of stress will stimulate your brain. That's good stress!

Heart disease

The connection between stress and heart attacks is well known. We've all heard of the middle-aged male executive who has a heart attack and then finally slows down and starts to take care of himself. Part of the reason for this effect is that stress raises adrenaline, which increases blood pressure and heart rate. This places more of a demand on the heart and circulatory system, increasing your risk for either a heart attack or, eventually, heart failure.

But cortisol and the HPA axis also influence heart health. A study in 2006 showed that men with the flattest cortisol curve were the most likely to have calcium buildup in their coronary arteries.[24] Having a flat cortisol curve indicated a significant stress load, and your HPA axis isn't responding normally. Somehow this affects the coronary arteries.

As we've mentioned, stress increases glucose, which contributes to blood vessel inflammation. We used to think heart attacks happened simply because your blood vessel slowly built up a blockage over time, and at some point it got so bad it clogged off. We now know that inflammation in the wall of the blood vessel is key to having a heart attack. You don't even really need a big blockage to have a heart attack. Inflammation all by itself can do this.

We also can't forget that stress causes people to do things that raise their cardiac risk, such as smoking, not exercising, and eating poorly. Stress is simply not good for heart health.

Digestive Issues

Stress most definitely affects digestion. In functional medicine, we talk about the *gut-brain connection*. This means when your brain isn't working right, you are more likely to have gastrointestinal issues. It also goes the other way: if your gut is inflamed and causing problems, your brain won't get the right nutrients and won't work optimally.

We used to talk about stress-induced ulcers, especially years ago before we had proton-pump inhibitors (like omeprazole). It turns out that most ulcers are caused by anti-inflammatory medications or an infection called

Helicobacter pylori, not so much from psychological stress. But stress can affect digestion in many ways, including thinning the normal mucosal barrier in your stomach that prevents the acid from eating through your stomach. Stress can also loosen the lower esophageal sphincter (LES), which is opening from the esophagus into the stomach. When the LES relaxes, stomach acid can reflux up, causing heartburn.

Just a note on taking antacids like esomeprazole and omeprazole (proton pump inhibitors, or PPIs): they aren't good for you! You may not even know that they aren't FDA approved for long term use. Your stomach was designed to be a holding tank full of battery acid. It's supposed to be the place where chewed up food starts being digested. The pepsin and hydrochloric acid breaks down proteins, which then go into the small intestine partially digested already. When you take a PPI like omeprazole, your stomach is mostly filled with water, not acid. Proteins are barely digested when they go into the small intestine, which then must work overtime to try to digest the food. You lose out on some amino acids, vitamins and minerals. PPIs are linked to deficiencies of vitamin B12, magnesium, calcium, and vitamin C. If you take them, try to wean off them by good nutrition, sleep, exercise, and stress management.

What I think is an even bigger stress problem in the gut is *leaky gut*. The technical term is "intestinal hyperpermeability," but we all call it leaky gut. Because of stress, toxins, or some foods, the normally tight junctions between cells become wide open and leaky. This allows undigested food or toxins to sneak into the blood vessels directly, instead of going through the cell like it's supposed to. It's like a bad guy with a weapon sneaking around the line at the airport and getting into the terminal without going through security. Not a good thing. Proteins or toxins gets into your blood stream and can damage cells anywhere in the body. This can cause the lining of the gut to get red and sore, if you could see it. Abdominal pain, bloating, diarrhea, or constipation result. Your digestion is now all messed up. What do we call it? Irritable bowel syndrome, or IBS.

I frankly hate the term IBS. People think it's an actual diagnosis. Far from it . . . it only describes a cluster of symptoms. Ask any gastroenterologist what is causing IBS and he or she will almost certainly say that they don't know. The three biggest factors causing IBS are stress, toxins, and eating the wrong food for your body. If you detox chemicals, pesticides and other bad stuff out of your body, only eat healthy organic whole foods that are right for you and reduce your stress, I virtually guarantee your gut inflammation will improve.

Fibromyalgia and Chronic Fatigue Syndrome

Fibromyalgia is characterized by widespread, unexplained pain, usually with significant fatigue and depression. For years, we had no idea what caused it, while noting a strong correlation with mood disorders. While stress clearly worsens the symptoms of fibromyalgia, it is not clear whether stress makes the pain worse or if it reduces one's ability to deal with the pain. But, either way, stress makes living with fibromyalgia more difficult. As many health care professionals felt it was all psychosomatic, i.e. a weakness in personality or a subconscious need to be sick, fibromyalgia has somewhat of a stigma to this day.

What is interesting is that we often see low cortisol levels in fibromyalgia. This makes sense if you consider most of these people are just exhausted all the time. One theory is that chronic stress is a factor in getting fibromyalgia, or at least a trigger.

We have realized that a common finding in fibromyalgia is that the low cortisol levels are from low CRH (corticotropin releasing hormone). The hypothalamus just doesn't make enough CRH, so the pituitary doesn't make as much ACTH, and the result that there is less cortisol made. Something going on in the brain is causing lower hypothalamus function.

A very intriguing connection we have made in the past few years is that fibromyalgia is often exactly like the symptoms of mold illness, chronic Lyme disease, long COVID or other chronic viral infections that are very difficult to diagnose. Common features of all of these are chronic fatigue, depression, joint and muscle pain, and brain fog. Inflammation is the common factor. All of them can cause inflammation in your brain.

Your hypothalamus is then suppressed, so you have less cortisol and low sex hormones. Low cortisol and CRH in fibromyalgia really may be one of these other diseases of abnormal immune response.

Miscellaneous

There are a lot of other symptoms and diseases that can be worsened by stress: eczema, psoriasis, arthritis, hair loss, cravings for sweet or salty foods, muscle tightness, headaches, low blood pressure, dizziness, overactive bladder, PMS, infertility. In essence, stress can make pretty much anything worse.

Spiritual Effects

Chronic stress is very dangerous, because it gets harder to respond in a positive, strong, faith-filled way. We all know how disheartening it is when a negative situation just doesn't change. It's very easy to lose hope.

When you have a negative outlook, it is easy to stop believing. This can lead to more depression, irritability, and anxiety, because you stop trusting God. You don't see God's purpose, so you think you've been wronged. You can easily get bitter, thinking you don't deserve what you're getting. You stop talking to God, shying away from His Word and avoiding church. Spiritual death has happened to many after chronic stress begins.

Satan would like nothing better than to discourage you and steal your faith. But without faith, you'll never have a true relationship with God. "Without faith, it is impossible to please Him, for he who comes to God must believe that He is, and that He is a rewarder of those who diligently seek Him" (Hebrews 11:6). Faith is believing that God is who He says He is and that He is able to take care of our every need. When you are mired in the misery of your own problems, you aren't looking to your Savior, and you really aren't any good to Him in advancing the Kingdom. Satan uses stress as his major weapon to get us off course in our walk with God. "Be sober, be vigilant; because your adversary the devil walks about like a roaring lion, seeking whom he may devour. Resist him, steadfast in the faith" (I Peter 5:8-9). He can throw stress at us all day long, but if we are on guard and prepared, we can use our faith to respond in a positive way.

Now that we've talked about all the devastating things that can happen with chronic stress, let's take a step back and consider the question: *What can we do about it?* There is a big difference between how helpless and powerless we sometimes feel when we go through stress and how powerful we truly are to use it for good.

Always remember that some stress is good for you. If you don't have any stress, how are you going to get stronger or better? Athletes train and fail so that they can get stronger. Artists have to fail in order to improve and succeed. Doctors go through years of school and residency to grow in knowledge and experience. Would you want a surgeon operating on you who never had to work through the night or deal with emergency situations? Would you want your attorney representing you if he or she had never been to court? Stress makes us better. But only if you handle it right.

When stress comes on, the first step is to recognize it. We then need to do an honest assessment of what we have control over, and then we need to develop a strategic plan. Let's look at how to get started.

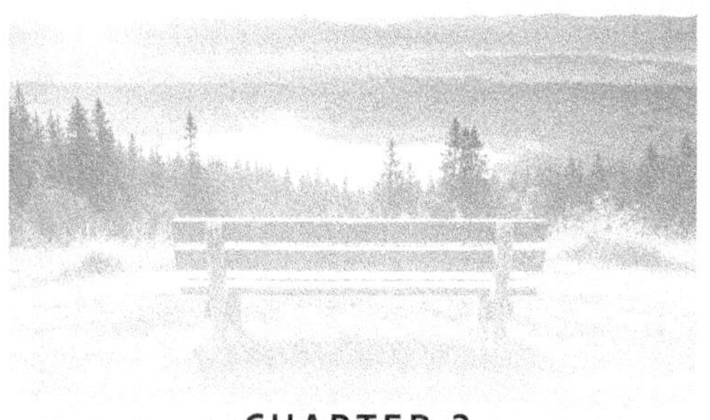

CHAPTER 3

How to Assess Physical Effect of Stress

If you have read this far, you're probably wondering how much stress is affecting your body. Start by discussing this with your physician. Get a good assessment from your doctor. He or she will check your blood pressure, do an examination, and may do standard bloodwork. This will pick up obvious things like high blood pressure, diabetes, a heart rhythm issue, or other things. However, you need to consider more in-depth testing as well.

Despite having good intentions for your health, most primary care physicians are not able or willing to do further testing. This is partly because they simply haven't had additional training in functional medicine. If they don't understand the value in this testing, they just won't do it. Also, most physicians are in very busy insurance-based clinics where they only have about ten-fifteen minutes for each patient visit. They have an enormous amount of work to do, including entering everything in the computer system, so they really don't have time to have a leisurely chat with you about the things you have researched or would like them to do. Finally, some physicians feel challenged by requests for alternative tests, and they will flat out refuse and tell you that those tests are unnecessary.

Be prepared for a less-than-optimal response, but it is always good to at least start with your doctor and get some testing done. The next step would be to see a functional medicine or integrative medicine practitioner. Many of us are MDs or DOs, but there are a lot of PAs and NPs doing functional medicine as well. Look for someone who has been doing functional medicine for more than a few years. It's a complex field, and it takes a while to get a handle on it. You can also consider seeing a naturopathic doctor, or ND. While in most states they cannot prescribe any medications, they are experts in functional medicine and can do the same testing we do, and they are experts at using supplements and dietary approaches.

Please note that, while there are some labs that offer functional testing online, it is always best to have a practitioner guide you to the exact testing that is most worthwhile for you. Then he or she can help you with the treatment needed based on the results.

Adrenals and Cortisol

Checking your cortisol levels is easy, but it is not something most doctors have ever done. While it is possible to check cortisol in your morning bloodwork, what we really want is four or five cortisol levels spaced out through the day. Getting your blood drawn all day long isn't very practical.

I prefer to check cortisol in urine or saliva throughout the day. This is painless and easy to do. Saliva has been used for years to check cortisol and sex hormones. All you have to do is spit in a plastic tube, which takes about ten-fifteen minutes, every four hours or so. We get a cortisol curve, which typically looks like this:

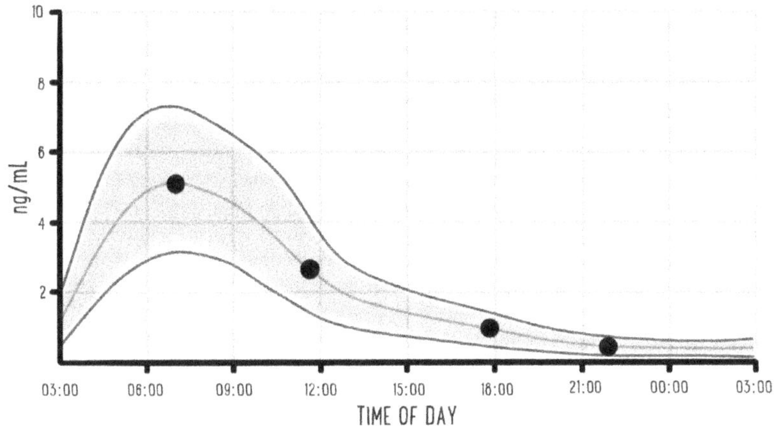

NORMAL SALIVA CORTISOL CURVE
Used with permission from ZRT Laboratory

You can also check cortisol in urine. You will typically collect four or five samples at different times, and then you get a cortisol curve:

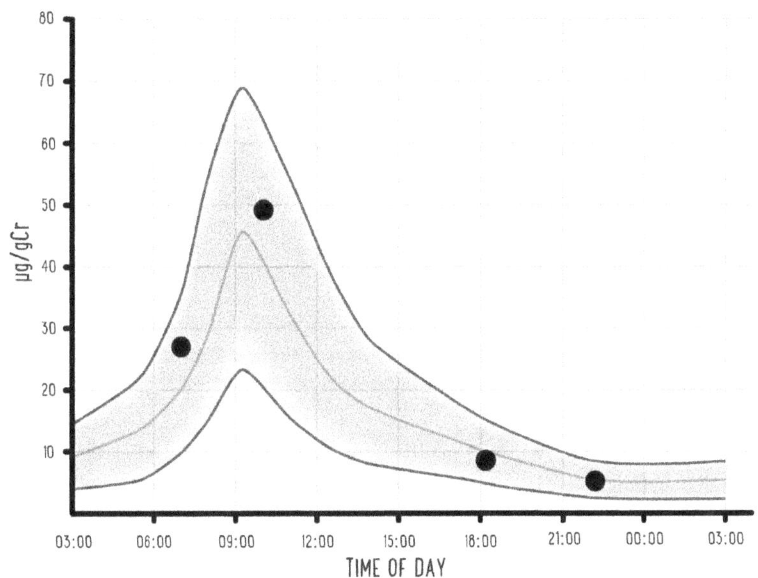

NORMAL URINE CORTISOL CURVE
Used with permission from ZRT Laboratory

This curve shows a modest rise in cortisol between the first two samples of the day. Your cortisol production should go up by about 50 percent the first hour you are awake. This is called the cortisol awakening response and indicates normal adrenal capacity to deal with the stress of the day.

A common unhealthy pattern is high cortisol through the whole day. Working out or a moderately stressful event can cause your cortisol to go up for a few hours, but if it comes back down to normal quickly, that isn't bad for you. But when it is high all day, it's not good for you and can cause you to feel anxious, irritable, or just plain stressed. It makes it hard to unwind and relax, especially at the end of the day. High cortisol in the evening is correlated with insomnia and poor sleep. It will destroy your peace and make it very difficult to enjoy all the good things you have in life. "The thief does not come except to steal, and to kill, and to destroy" (John 10:10).

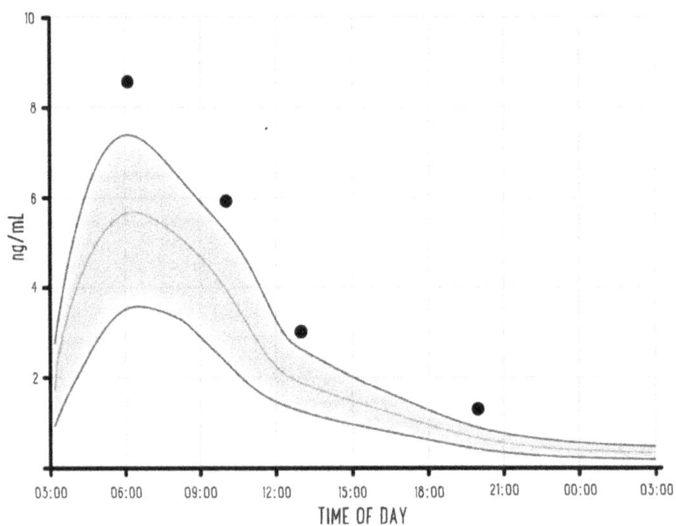

HIGH CORTISOL CURVE
Used with permission by ZRT Laboratory

This pattern is common early on in a stressful period in life. If your cortisol levels run high beyond the stressful period, your challenge is to learn how not to overreact to negative thoughts and events. You need to work on stress reduction techniques to bring peace back into your life.

If stress continues long-term, eventually your cortisol levels will drop and be lower than normal. If you have a low, flat curve, you aren't making enough cortisol, so you tend to be tired and won't handle stress well. You feel burned out. This usually indicates that your system is overall tired, and the stress is causing serious damage.

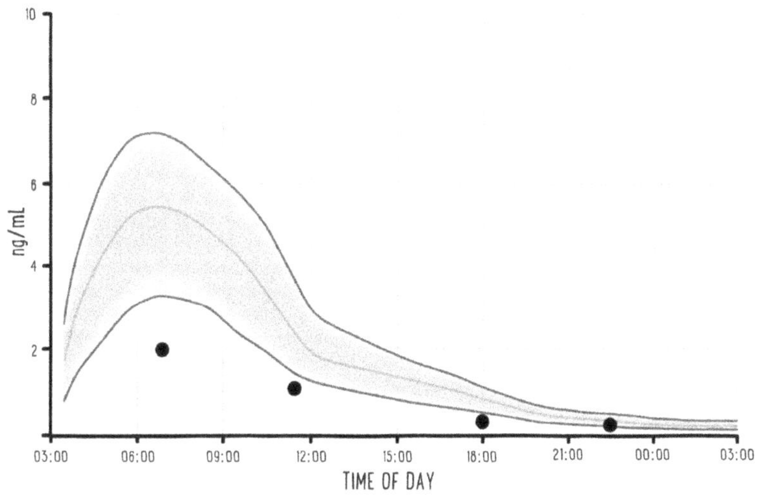

LOW CORTISOL CURVE
Used with permission by ZRT Laboratory

The other thing to look for is whether you have a normal cortisol awakening response to begin with. Your cortisol levels may all be normal through the day, but if your cortisol doesn't increase the first few hours of the day, your HPA axis is not responding normally. Flat curves have been associated with poorer cognitive function, PTSD, and blood vessel stiffness.[25]

Looking at your cortisol curve can be very insightful. It doesn't always match how you feel, but it's amazing how often it does. I tell my patients it is a strong signal that stress is affecting you physically and medically, and it isn't just an emotion or a thought in your brain. It is hurting your body and having affects you probably aren't aware of. Like the red light on your dashboard showing "check engine," you need to evaluate your stress and your responses.

Brain Health

How can you tell if your brain is being affected by stress? Just ask a family member. They will almost certainly tell you if you are stressed! Beyond that, there are in-depth medical cognitive tests that can be done, but they are usually not necessary.

The first thing you can evaluate is your sleep. When you are stressed, your sleep is often the first thing to suffer. Ask yourself:

> » How quickly do you fall asleep?
>
> » Do you routinely get at least seven hours of sleep?
>
> » Do you wake up for more than ten minutes in the night?
>
> » Do you wake up with a dry, sore throat or aches and pains?
>
> » Are you able to wake up and not be groggy within an hour?

If you are having any problems getting a good night sleep, your brain is being affected and is not healthy.

The second thing that evaluates how healthy your brain is, are your moods. Again, ask yourself:

> » Do you feel joy most days?
>
> » Do you enjoy your work?
>
> » Are you invigorated by something (either work or a hobby)?
>
> » Are you so passionate about something that you love to share it with others?
>
> » Do you feel satisfaction in a job well done?
>
> » Do you enjoy being with others or do they mostly annoy you?
>
> » Do you see all the things wrong with your life, or do you see the blessings?

Good emotional health typically means your brain is relatively unaffected by stress. Conversely, people who have a lot of brain inflammation from brain diseases often have mood disorders. We see this often in people with fibromyalgia, CIRS, or even menopause. These people tend to have significant mood swings from anxiety to depression to just simply irritability and brain fog. This can happen in certain types of dementia, as well.

But thank goodness, it doesn't necessarily have to be that way! Have you ever known someone fighting cancer who had the sweetest spirit and was still a joy to others? I have been so privileged to take care of patients who chose to have a grateful heart even in their last days. They always thanked me for my care, even though I felt like I really couldn't do much for them. But relieving their symptoms was so appreciated by them. I remember Patty, dying of ALS, thanking me for making a house call. Rob fought his prostate cancer for several years. We thought we had it licked, but it came back with a vengeance. He was so easy to take care of medically, but he always thanked me profusely. I remember Julia, who refused to treat her tangerine-sized breast tumor. I begged her to see a surgeon, but she insisted on trusting God to heal her. She wanted to treat it naturally. She continued to refuse any traditional therapy, but she greatly appreciated that I respected her wish to use alternative treatments. Even while she was dying, she had such amazing joy.

But I've experienced the opposite, too. I have had so many patients with basically nothing wrong with them except normal stress, but a lot of them were bitter, needy people. All I could do was prescribe antidepressants and try to encourage them to get counseling, get some exercise, and the like. But they insisted on wallowing in their minor complaints. Frank was in his early fifties with diabetes and hypertension but only on a few medications. His labs were always good, but he always had a complaint. Often it was his sinuses, sometimes mild back pain, and once it was a very minor elevation in his liver tests (his terrible diet caused a condition called *fatty liver*). Every one of those visits took me thirty to forty minutes to reassure him that he wasn't dying. His self-absorption was so sad. He gave absolutely no joy to anyone he worked with, and he had few friends. And he always sucked energy from me. Yes, it was my job, but don't you want to be the kind of person to give joy and lift other people up?

We'll talk about psychological and spiritual strategies to lift your mood later. But just know that if you are grumpy and depressed, your brain is definitely not healthy. And it probably is affecting more than your mood: you probably aren't thinking as clearly as you should be, you are more distractible, and your memory isn't as sharp. Good brain health is essential.

The third thing to assess regarding brain health is cognitive functions. How sharp is your mind? How good is your memory? Subtle changes may not be easy for us to recognize in ourselves. Even when we do admit we aren't as sharp, we tend to underestimate how bad it is. We learn to compensate for it.

Many years ago, I had a very stressful few years. My husband and I were not getting along very well, our young kids were acting up a lot, Daniel's struggles were becoming more visible and harder to manage, and to top it all off, we were dirt poor. I went to work to escape the stress at home, but work was just as stressful, because I was basically losing money instead of making it. (I started a solo practice in a rural area and insurance companies didn't pay very well at all.) I remember that, with the depression and irritability came a notable drop in my ability to focus. I wasn't making mistakes at work, but I was unfocused, and it was a huge effort to see a complex patient. I had to address five or six conditions, review labs, renew meds, and deal with new issues or complications. What should have been easy was a monumental task. Multiply that by twenty people in a day, and my brain was pretty much fried. I forgot to do the extra things like stopping for eggs on the way home or calling my mother to check on her. I also began stumbling over my words. My daughter used to laugh at me, because I would combine two words into one. My brain couldn't decide between coat and jacket, so it figured *coacket* was good enough.

When you have chronic stress, your brain neurons just don't connect quite as well as they are supposed to. It's like getting up at three a.m. and trying to do algebra problems. You can get by, and you'll fool a lot of people, but don't fool yourself by thinking it's not a big deal. It is. You were designed to be smart, think quickly, and remember well.

Sex Hormones

How do you know if your sex hormones are affected by stress? There are a lot of different ways we can check these hormones. We can look for them in venous blood, saliva, capillary blood (by finger prick), and urine. There are pros and cons of each type of hormone test, and they differ in men and women.

For women, blood is often used, but many of us find it to be a bit less useful as the other methods. That's because there is a wide range for these hormones, and they don't always match symptoms. For example, estradiol (the main form of estrogen) in blood for cycling women can normally be anywhere from 12–498 pg/ml in one common lab. It is low the first ten days of the cycle, then peaks around ovulation, then stays middle of the range for a while then comes down. If a woman has irregular cycles, what does it mean if the estradiol is 40? Is that normal or low? What if it's 370? Is that okay or too high? It can be hard to match blood levels with symptoms. For example, low estrogen often causes hot flashes and brain fog. If your estradiol is 70, is that too low for you and you need it raised? Or is it totally fine and your symptoms are from something else? Very difficult to know. Once women go on hormone therapy at menopause, however, we do use blood testing more often, as there is no cycling to try to figure out.

Salivary testing of hormones has been used for years. There are several advantages to saliva testing. Firstly, it is easy to do at home, and it doesn't hurt. Secondly, it measures the free portion of hormone, not the total, so it is measuring only the biologically active form of the hormone. Thirdly, the levels in saliva have a narrow reference range. For example, we like to see estradiol from one-five or so in saliva. If it comes back nine, it's probably too high. Likewise, a level of 0.2 is probably going to give you hot flashes. We know then to increase your estrogen dose.

Urine is another interesting way to look at sex hormones. It turns out that there are a lot of different forms of testosterone, estrogen and progesterone that we can analyze in the urine. We can get a lot of information about how your body is processing your hormones and how they are being eliminated. For example, certain androgens (testosterone, DHEA and several others) are associated with acne and facial hair. If your testosterone is causing these annoying side effects, sometimes we can figure out why and then attempt to block these androgens with supplements or medications. We also can assess various metabolites of estrogen, which tells us if you are detoxing correctly.

There are differences in these methods that we providers learn with experience. For example, creams don't raise blood levels as much as pills or injectables. Blood levels for estrogen, progesterone, and testosterone vary a lot based on whether you are on a pill form, a cream, or pellets. Sometimes, blood levels won't go up at all on a cream, but it depends on which hormone and the dose. I find that urine is a better way to assess estrogen therapy, as we can check different types of estrogens, which gives us a better picture of your overall total estrogens levels and we can see how your body is detoxing them.

Blood tests are quick and easy, but urine or saliva often gives us more information. I always do urine testing on my new patients because it includes the cortisol curve we have talked about. You just can't get that from bloodwork alone. Each provider who is experienced in bioidentical hormone replacement therapy (BHRT) will have his or her own preferences on testing. But the more you know, the better you can discuss it with him or her.

Once again, please do not be surprised if your primary care physician refuses to check your hormones. They simply are not trained to do so. Find a good provider who is experienced in BHRT.

Thyroid Hormone

As I mentioned in the last chapter, thyroid function is often affected by stress, and symptoms of low thyroid can mimic stress. The thyroid gland makes thyroid hormone, which is like a gasoline additive. The gas is the nutrients you eat, but when you add a performance-enhancing additive, your fuel works a lot better. Thyroid hormone goes into a cell and drives its metabolism, creating energy.

Low thyroid levels, or hypothyroidism, causes fatigue, brain fog, constipation, unexplained weight gain, and fluid retention. You feel like you're moving through thickening cement. Fortunately, any physician can check your thyroid levels. The main test done is TSH, and it is a pretty good screening tool.

TSH is a little confusing to some. It stands for Thyroid Stimulating Hormone. It is made in the pituitary, and it technically isn't a thyroid hormone. Its job is to go to the thyroid, and it tells it to make more thyroid hormone. Then the thyroid makes T3 and T4, the actual thyroid hormones. TSH is inversely related to T3 and T4. When your thyroid gets sluggish and your thyroid hormones levels are low, your TSH will be high. The best analogy is that you are the pituitary and your kids are the thyroid. They are sitting on the couch playing video games, doing absolutely nothing useful, so you start telling at them to get up and play outside. They still are doing nothing, so you eventually end up yelling to get their attention. The TSH signal goes up because the thyroid is lazy and not doing its job.

The opposite is also true. When your thyroid is overactive (hyperthyroidism), the TSH signal from the pituitary goes down. If you are on too high of a thyroid dose, your TSH goes way down and will be suppressed.

Opinions vary on the optimal TSH range. While it should not be over 5 for most people, many of us in functional medicine like to see it under 2.5 to 3. The lower limit is usually around 0.4. If your TSH is 0.4-3.0, you are less likely to have a significant thyroid issue. Many primary care physicians will say that a TSH of 3.5 to 4.9 is normal. While it technically is in the normal range printed on the lab results, I believe it's a sign that something isn't quite right in the thyroid.

Another situation usually missed by primary care physicians is if you are a poor converter. This is common when stress is affecting your thyroid hormone production. Let's look at thyroid hormones in a little more detail.

TSH causes the thyroid to make thyroid hormone, which is about 80 percent T4 and about 20 percent T3.

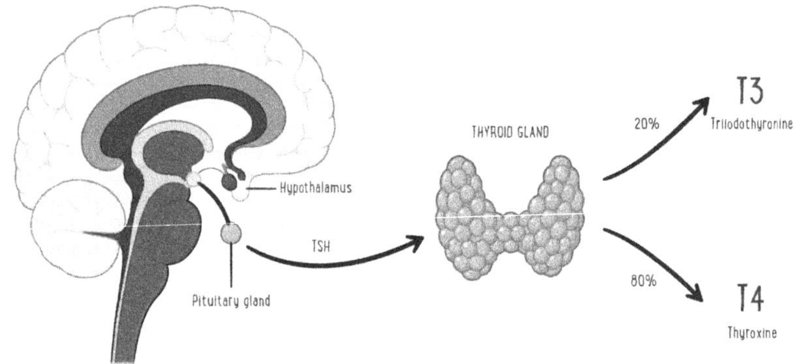

TSH causes the thyroid to make thyroid hormone,
which is about 80 percent T4 and about 20 percent T3.

T4 and T3 refer to the total amount of those hormones. However, an even better lab test is free T3 and free T4, called fT4 and fT3. This is the small percentage of T3 and T4 that are free and not bound up to proteins, so they are the biologically active part that we really want to look at. (Protein bound hormone just circulates around, but doesn't do much unless it detaches from the protein.)

The fT4 that is made and released goes out into the body, where an enzyme has to convert it to fT3. Free T3 is really the ultimate powerhouse form that goes into the cells and revs up their metabolism. So fT4 is important, but arguably fT3 is even more important. But the conversion of fT4 to fT3 can go wrong with stress.

You need certain nutrients for this conversion: vitamin A, vitamin C, vitamin E and zinc. If you don't have enough of any of these, your fT4 will go down the other pathway, to the form called reverse T3, or rT3. In the last chapter, I called this the dud form. It looks like fT3, but the molecule is the reverse image. It's like trying to use your left hand to shake someone's outstretched right hand. It looks identical, but it is a mirror image, so it doesn't fit!

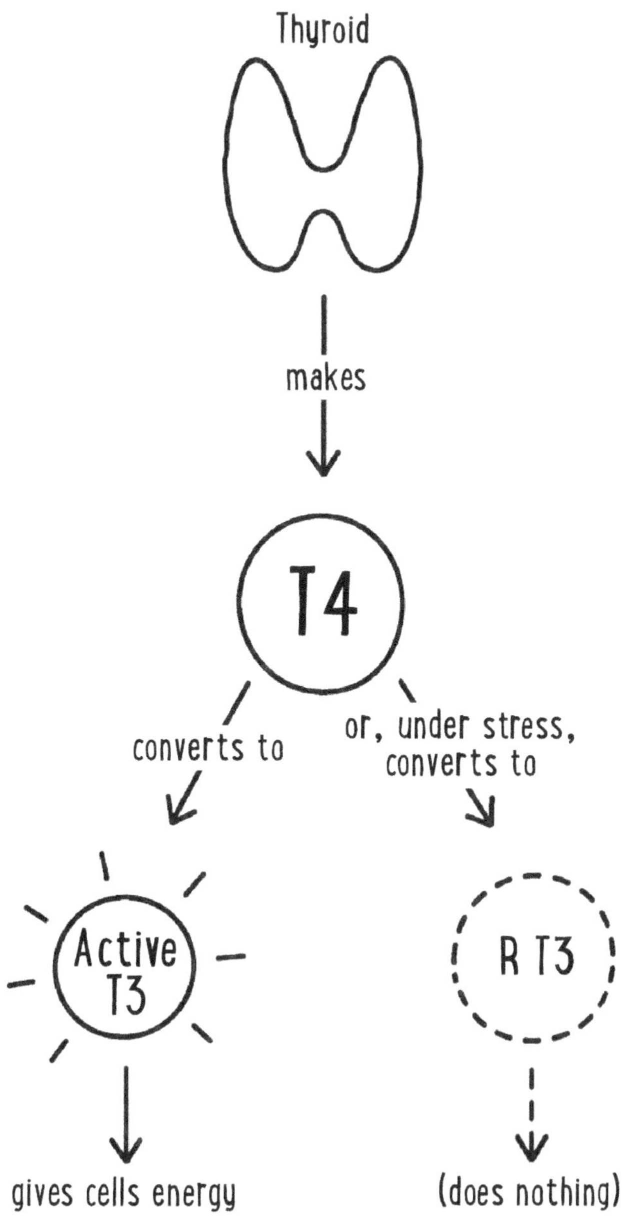

T4 to T3 conversion.

In addition to nutrient deficiency, stress is a big reason for this. Stress causes a shift, so a lot more of your fT4 becomes rT3 and less becomes fT3. Then your doctor tells you that your TSH is fine. But you still are exhausted, constipated, and unable to lose weight. But no one looked at your fT3. Almost any lab can check fT4, fT3 and rT3 but most doctors (even endocrinologists) will tell you there isn't any reason to check them. They are wrong. I see people all the time with a normal TSH and normal fT4, but low normal T3 and elevated rT3. It's because of stress. The solution? Use supplements to support the conversion to fT3, use thyroid hormone when necessary, and reduce the stress response.

Gut Health

Another way we know stress is affecting you physically is if you have digestive issues. Have you ever said "I can feel it in my gut" or been nauseated thinking about a stressful situation? Literature is full of references to gastrointestinal function related to emotions. Isaiah even said, "My stomach aches and burns with pain. Sharp pangs of anguish are upon me, like those of a woman in labor" (Isaiah 21:3 NLT).

Digestion is so closely tied with stress or the lack thereof. When you have a stressful event coming up, you may stress eat, or you may lose your appetite completely. I used to lose my appetite before big tests in medical school or first days on a new rotation in the hospital. Then after the test, I would be ravenous and pig out! High stress releases adrenaline (epinephrine), which tends to reduce appetite. This is our way of being ready for the attack. If an antelope just ate a five-course meal, how well would he run away from the lion?

In the short term, GI symptoms are simply annoying. But when you have stress day after day, it is likely to make things much worse. You get what we call *leaky gut*. As explained earlier, cortisol weakens the "tight junctions" between gut cells, widening them up. Bad stuff crosses through and gets into the bloodstream causing a lot of problems.

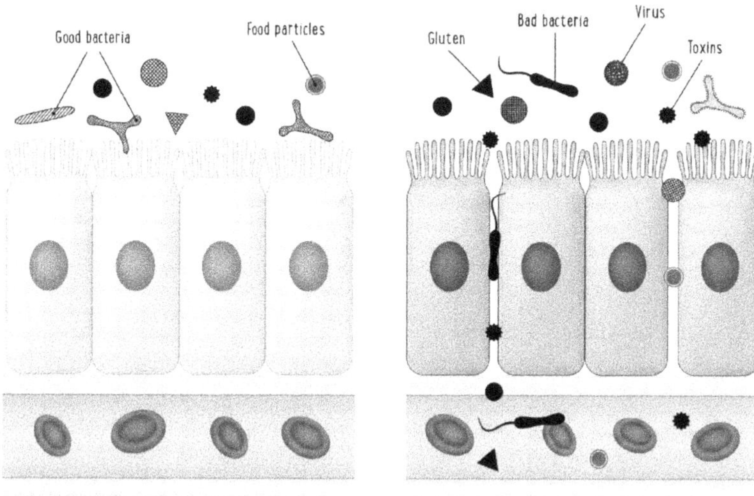

LEAKY GUT

Although there is a range of normal bowel movements, here are some things that are not normal:

>> Not having at least one bowel movement a day

>> Having more than five or six in a day

>> Loose (unformed) stools

>> Passing significant gas

>> Blood or mucus with bowel movements

>> Abdominal pain with bowel movements

There are several ways to test your gut to see how healthy it is. However, many of these specific tests are not done by most primary care physicians or even gastroenterologists. In my experience, gastroenterologists are somewhat limited in their treatment of the root cause beneath common symptoms. While they do diagnose and treat inflammatory bowel disease and even cancer and can perform endoscopies, it often seems that they do not have the knowledge to address the root causes of digestive issues.

Functional testing includes stool analysis as well as looking for food sensitivities. There are now labs doing stool testing for DNA analysis of the many types of bacteria that live inside of you, called your microbiome. The research on the microbiome is just fascinating. You have trillions of bacteria in your gut that you live in harmony with, or at least you're supposed to. But stress, antibiotics, and toxins can destroy the good bacteria. Then you get more of the bad bacteria. Did you know some bacteria species have been linked to certain autoimmune diseases? Some are linked to obesity and diabetes. We are learning new things from this research every day. If you have dysbiosis, or a change in your gut bacteria, you should treat it. It usually means you need to tweak your diet, and you need a probiotic with other supplements to heal your gut. Stool testing is an easy way to find out.

Stool testing also looks for markers of inflammation, blood, and markers of abnormal digestion. We can tell a lot about your gut health with a small sample. A test can determine how well you are absorbing food, if you are inflamed, if you have leaky gut, if you have enough good bacteria, if you have too many bad bacteria, and even if you have a parasite.

I also frequently test for food sensitivities to see if there are some healthy foods you may be eating that are not the right thing for your body right now. I like labs that check not only for antibodies to a certain food but also signs of immune complex formation with antibodies. Just having an antibody may or may not be associated with actual inflammation. Sometimes it means you eat that food regularly, and you have adapted to it. However, if the antibodies are part of an immune complex, this indicates you have triggered both the innate and adaptive immune systems, so it is much more concerning.

Most integrative practitioners recommend an elimination diet for anyone with GI symptoms. This is an alternative to food sensitivity testing, and, as I like to say, costs you zero dollars. Most elimination diets remove wheat, dairy, soy, corn, eggs, nuts, and sugar for few weeks. This often helps quite a bit and is easy to do on your own without a practitioner. But if you have already removed those foods from your diet and you still have symptoms, you should see if your immune system has been triggered by any of the healthy foods you have been eating.

It's amazing how often this testing shows something that is really a source of inflammation. Shockingly, it could be green pepper, vanilla, apples, asparagus, coffee, chicken, or almonds. These tests are looking for food that we otherwise would assume is very healthy for you. You would never know these foods were a problem for you unless you test! These sensitivities have to do with a different pathway in the immune system than typical food allergies. Food allergies are often shrimp or peanut, and allergies cause difficulty breathing, asthma, or hives. Sensitivities are not allergic reactions *per se*, but they cause irritation in the gut, which causes a wide variety of symptoms. I have seen people eliminate all sorts of digestive problems, as well as headaches, rashes, and joint pain, when they eliminate the foods that their body was sensitive to.

The lab I use for food sensitivity testing also tests for a reaction to two things called zonulin and occludin. These are proteins found in the tight junctions of the gut lining. If you have leaky gut, your immune system will react to them. If your test is positive, it means your food sensitivities are significant, you have leaky gut, and it's time to get your gut healed.

CHAPTER 4

Nutritional Strategies for Healing

I like to talk about nutrition before we talk about medical things like supplements and medications. You might be thinking, come on, I know how to eat healthy. Tell me what I can take! But you would be missing the most important thing here. You are what you eat! There is just such tremendous power in eating healthy. You simply cannot eat a poor diet and then expect to take a pill to somehow compensate for a lack of nutrition. Even gut-healing supplements will not work very well if you are still eating food that is causing inflammation.

Nutrition is consuming the necessary nutrients for our cells to function. Most Americans are deficient in the following:

- » Magnesium
- » Calcium
- » Vitamin D
- » Vitamin E
- » Folate
- » Vitamin A

The biggest issue is that people eat too many foods that are rich in sugar and calories but are low in nutrients. They are feeding emotional needs with sugar and fat but starving their cells of the nutrients they need.

Consider the following diet:

- » **Breakfast:** Cereal with non-organic, low-fat milk
- » **Lunch:** Sandwich with processed lunch meat and chips
- » **Supper:** Spaghetti and garlic bread, salad with ranch dressing and croutons

This diet is high in starchy carbohydrates, low in protein and low in fiber. It also is high is vegetable oils and low in healthy fats. Some people might argue that those meals aren't that bad. You're right; you could be eating a doughnut for breakfast and fast food for lunch. Many people do! But those choices are nutritionally lacking for the following reasons:

- » **Breakfast:** all carbs, virtually no protein, no healthy fats
- » **Lunch:** refined flour, full of carbs, preservatives and nitrites, trans fats in chips.
- » **Supper:** mostly refined flour full of carbs, not a lot of protein and fats are from seed oil.

Moving past macronutrients, how many vitamins and minerals do you think you're getting? Very few. We all should strive to get five to ten servings of fruits and vegetables a day. Most Americans get zero to two! Fruits and veggies, especially organic, are a rich source of vitamins, minerals and phytonutrients. They are full of nutrients and fiber but do not cause a rapid rise in glucose like starches do. Their fiber helps fill you up and keeps you full without your energy going up and down. It's amazing how many nutrients are in fruits and vegetables. You just can't get these in a french fry. My question to you is: How on earth do you expect your brain, your emotions, and your body to be stress resilient when you are starving your cells of badly needed nutrients? It just won't work.

When you buy your produce, try to get organic as much as you can. There are lists called "The Dirty Dozen" and "The Clean Fifteen" put out periodically by the Environmental Working Group. This is a list of the fruits and vegetables that have the most pesticides and herbicides in them, so these are the ones you should always try to buy organic. For example, strawberries, spinach, kale and apples should be organic. "The Clean Fifteen" are things like avocado, cabbage, cauliflower and broccoli which usually are clean, so you can skip the organic varieties.[26]

Stress eating is the total opposite of healthy eating. I totally understand stress eating, though. It sure does make you feel better right away! I tell everyone the only way I got through the long days of medical school was to reward myself at ten or eleven at night with a huge bowl of ice cream. I'm talking four or five scoops, with chocolate sauce and, sometimes, whipped cream. Boy, did that taste good! But then an hour later I totally crashed, felt fat and bloated, and collapsed into bed. Not a good long-term strategy.

We now know that eating sugar hits the same receptors in the brain that some drugs do. You get a surge of dopamine, the neurotransmitter associated with reward and pleasure. It really does make your brain feel better. But it is short lived and very damaging. Eating starches or sugar just keeps feeding the monster. Eating sugary foods is terrible for your stress resilience. It spikes your blood glucose up within minutes. But that causes your pancreas to release insulin. Insulin's job is to go out into the bloodstream, grab on to glucose, and pull it into the cells. The problem with this is that too much insulin makes you tired and gives you brain fog. I often have patients who complain about mid-afternoon fatigue. Quite often it is because they eat too many carbohydrates for lunch. This is from the surge in insulin, which makes you sleepy. I call it a *carb crash*. About an hour after eating too much sugar, you are in a total brain fog and falling asleep. This also affects your moods. You may overreact to things emotionally and make poor decisions. You basically can make yourself miserable and it is unnecessary.

Sugar is worth examining further. We have all heard "sugar is bad." That is mostly true, but there are different kinds of sugar. Think about nutrition up until about one hundred years ago. The amount of sugar the average person ate in in the early 1900s was about 15–30 g/day. Now it is over 100 g/day![27] We have so many high sugar, super sweet foods available to us, and many of us were raised to eat sugar cereal for breakfast, drink Kool-Aid®, and eat cookies and Twinkies® for dessert. We have become desensitized to sugar. Try eliminating soda for a month, then take a sip. You will be stunned how sweet it is!

Make it your goal to enjoy fruit as your dessert. A bowl of berries or a ripe peach should give you joy and satisfy you. I promise you that you will feel so much better after a good piece of fruit than after eating a sugary dessert. One more thing about sugar—don't drink it! Sugar is so easy to guzzle when it is in tea, soda or juice. Drinking eight ounces of orange juice contains the same sugar as two average-sized chocolate chip cookies. Don't fool yourself into thinking fruit juice is healthy. It is all the sugar and none of the fiber found in the fruit. Eat an orange or an apple instead of drinking it. Resist the sweets; you'll have much more steady energy.

Eat a diet full of healthy protein sources and good fats, with some carbs that don't turn into sugar very fast. Quinoa, brown rice, sweet potatoes, and legumes are healthy in the right quantities. They have fiber, and their starches turn into sugar more slowly than refined white flour or white potatoes. Skip the french fries and have beans or brown rice instead. Try making quinoa with veggies and seasonings. Slowly get the white flour and potatoes out of your diet. You'll feel better.

Gluten is inflammatory for a lot of us. No question. Wheat, which contains gluten, is simply indigestible for many people and causes a lot of gut inflammation. You may or may not have GI issues, but gluten can cause brain fog, joint pain, reflux, headaches, and weird rashes. If you're not feeling well, it's best to avoid gluten as much as possible.

Opinions vary regarding meat. From a medical standpoint, vegan and vegetarian diets are often too low in protein and too high in carbohydrates to be healthy. Women in particular who go vegan thinking they will lose weight are often sorely disappointed. Meat and eggs are great sources of protein. However, you need to be careful how you shop. Commercial beef is filled with omega-6 fatty acids and other fats, where grass fed beef is much higher in omega-3 fatty acids, which are much better for you. Free-range chicken likewise is nutritionally much better for you than typical commercially farmed chicken. Wild caught salmon and shrimp are better than farmed fish. I am a big proponent of incorporating clean sources of meat in your diet. Just be careful with how often you eat out: it rarely is cleanly sourced.

Fats are commonly thought of as "bad," especially saturated fats, such as those found in butter and red meat. But that isn't true. The food industry spent a lot of money in the past few decades trying to steer us toward vegetable (seed) oils. It turns out that oils like corn, canola, and soybean are harmful. Seed oils are inflammatory and are linked to chronic disease. They are high in omega-6 fats and not omega-3 fats which are anti-inflammatory. You're actually better off using organic butter than canola oil. Along that line, eggs are not bad for you. The whole idea that eating eggs raises your cholesterol was disproven years ago. But people still believe the myth that eating the small amount of cholesterol in an egg yolk will raise your blood level of cholesterol. It doesn't. Your blood level of cholesterol is controlled mostly by the amount and type of cholesterol your liver makes, as well as by the amount of carbohydrates and seed oils you eat. It's totally fine to eat organic, free-range eggs. They are a great source of nutrients, including choline, which supports memory and cognitive function.

Alcohol and caffeine can contribute to poor health. Many Americans jump start their energy with morning coffee. One or two cups is okay for most people, but more than that usually causes cortisol to go up. This is the same physical response as if you have stress, but it is from caffeine. I see patients every day who compensate for their fatigue with coffee. Those under high stress are only getting by. The stress raised their cortisol, then they typically crash with exhaustion, which requires coffee to get going in the morning. Coffee is not bad for you, but if you're using more than two cups to function, that's a signal you probably have a stress issue you need to address.

Millions of people also use alcohol to relax at the end of the day. I can't tell you how many women come to see me with mood swings and trouble losing weight, and they tell me they have a glass or two of wine every night to unwind. Alcohol is a toxin, remember? It damages the nerve transmission between cells in the brain. Then your liver must detoxify it and eliminate it. This can affect both your brain and your liver.

Matthew Walker explains in *Why We Sleep* how damaging alcohol is to sleep.[28] Many people say that alcohol helps them fall asleep. While this sometimes is true, what they are missing is that alcohol damages your sleep cycles. You will not spend enough time in non-REM, restorative sleep. Your sleep cycles will be more erratic. You will not wake up as refreshed. The help is just an illusion. Alcohol makes your sleep worse. When your sleep is consistently a problem, you gain weight, and your moods are affected. You are tired, and therefore less stress resilient the next day.

Aside from poor sleep, which can prevent weight loss, alcohol itself can make you fat. Its calories are from carbs, and they stop fat from burning. Even if you only have one or two glasses at night, it can shut down any fat burning that would have happened and move your metabolism more towards fat storage, thus preventing you from losing weight. Keep alcohol use infrequent and avoid it when you are stressed.

We probably don't need to talk much about junk food, because if it's in this category, we all know it's junk! But be aware that trans fats cause brain damage. These are a type of fat found in commercial baked goods like crackers, cookies, microwave popcorn, frozen desserts, frozen pizza, refrigerated dough products, doughnuts, and shortening. Trans fats get incorporated into the outer membrane of cells and permanently deform the cell membrane. Once they are in there, you can't get them out. When the cell membrane is distorted, the function of the cell is damaged. Cell damage like this in brain neurons is a form of brain damage. Trans fats are also terrible for your blood vessels and increase your risk for a heart attack. So just don't. God gave us amazing foods for nourishment. Don't substitute frozen waffles or pizza and wonder why you feel bad. A good rule of thumb for nutrition is to only eat foods that were foods 100 years ago. Coffee, eggs, produce, and meat were foods. But junk food was not!

I know that is it hard to change your diet! When I first found out that my irritable bowel symptoms were really gluten sensitivity, it was hard to accept. This was many years ago when gluten free products were hard to find, expensive, and didn't taste very good. But I did it because I quickly realized that eating a slice of pizza was totally not worth having abdominal pain for three days. I felt so much better when I cleaned up my diet and healed my gut. It is worth the effort!

Just because you are sensitive to certain foods right now does not mean that you will always be. Once you heal your gut, the lining of your intestine will return to normal and it is quite likely that you will be able to eat a lot of those foods again. You might not be able to eat them often, but a lot of food sensitivities do go away with time and some TLC.

Work with an integrative practitioner to assess your gut health and identify which foods might be an issue for you right now. Accept whatever you find and revise your diet. Focus on all the amazingly tasty foods you can tolerate, and don't focus on the ones you can't. Experiment with cooking. I am a big believer in looking up new recipes online for vegetables you may not eat often. For example, I hated Brussels sprouts growing up, as some of you may have. But that's because Mom boiled them. *Yuck!* I love to marinate them in a mix of olive oil, balsamic vinegar, lime, and some other spices, then I bake them in the oven. They turn out so yummy! I love crunching on the stray leaves that fall off and turn crispy as they bake. They are better than potato chips.

Try new meals that mix vegetables with meat, either in a stir fry, crock pot, or baking dish. There are endless possibilities for healthy, low carb meals made with delicious spices and seasonings. You will not find healthy cooking at most restaurants, but you can make your favorite meals with clean ingredients when you cook at home. Remember, God gave us plant foods for food. We read in Genesis, "And God said, 'See, I have given you every herb that yields seed which is on the face of all the earth, and every tree whose fruit yields seed; to you it shall be for food. Also, to every beast of the earth, to every bird of the air, and to everything that creeps on the earth, in which there is life, I have given every green herb for food'; and it was so. Then God saw everything that He had made, and indeed it was very good" (Gen 1:29–31).

Medical Strategies for Healing

Adrenals

Okay, so you checked your cortisol levels through the course of a day, and they are either too high or too low. You know you're stressed, and your cortisol levels prove it. Now what?

The first thing is to not stress over your cortisol curve. Don't put too much weight on the exact numbers that showed up on that day you tested. Many of us have shifted our approach to HPA axis dysfunction. We used to overanalyze the cortisol curve and use various targeted supplements. Supplements such as phosphatidylserine help lower elevated cortisol. I often had patients obsess over one or two of their cortisol levels on a test. They were very frustrated that we couldn't explain why it was high or low at that specific time. Sometimes it makes sense, but quite often it doesn't. Remember, your cortisol level is always changing. It's like your speed driving to work. Sometimes you might zip along at sixty mph, but sometimes it's only twenty-five mph, and at a stop light, it's zero. Keep the big picture in mind. One of your cortisol levels may be high or low, but if it doesn't correlate with how you typically feel at that time of an average day, don't worry too much about it. I tell my patients that we are looking at cortisol with a birds-eye view. Let's get the overall picture: are they mostly normal, are some of them high or are some low? That helps frame our approach.

It also can be frustrating when you take an adrenal supplement faithfully for months but then you don't see much improvement in your cortisol curve. Again, that's because the cortisol curve is not quite as black and white as we thought. Additionally, while supplements can be very helpful, they alone are usually not enough to fix the problem entirely.

Most quality supplement companies have several products for adrenal support or stress. These herbs are called "adaptogens" by medical professionals because they have been used for many years for stress resilience. These include:

- » Ashwagandha
- » Rhodiola
- » Skullcap
- » Eleuthero
- » American Ginseng
- » Schisandra
- » Licorice root
- » Phosphatidylserine
- » L-theanine
- » Green tea (has L-theanine in it naturally)
- » Magnolia bark and phellodendron
- » GABA
- » Adrenal glandulars
- » Nicotinamide riboside or nicotinamide adenine dinucleotide (NAD)

Most formulas have several ingredients that all work together. One alone usually isn't very helpful, but a good blend of several adaptogens can work wonders. Typically, they help you react less emotionally to stress. Things don't bother you quite as much. You are less likely to feel like punching a wall or yell at your kids. You don't feel as overwhelmed, and you can let things go more easily. You just don't feel your stress quite as emotionally, so you handle it better.

I recommend that you take your adrenal support supplement every day at the same time of day. If stress is significant, twice a day may be warranted. However, you should always discuss your situation with your provider to get his or her recommendations for your specific situation. They know the products and how they are best taken.

A few of these adaptogens are worth mentioning further. Ashwagandha is the mainstay of adaptogens. It is an Ayurvedic herb often found in these supplements. It helps many aspects of the stress response. Interestingly, it may work by reducing brain inflammation, which allows your HPA axis to heal. It benefits blood pressure and the immune system. There is data showing that ashwagandha reduces cortisol and perceived stress, as well as anxiety.[29]

If you have low cortisol or a flat-line curve, I recommend licorice root, which has glycyrrhizic acid as its main component. Note: Candy licorice doesn't have this; you have to use a high-quality supplement. Licorice inhibits the enzyme that breaks down cortisol, thereby increasing cortisol levels. However, licorice in higher doses can cause fluid retention. You should not take licorice if you have any heart or kidney disease or if you have high blood pressure.

For further support of low cortisol, adrenal glandulars are often used. With these you are ingesting small amounts of adrenal gland (typically bovine) which has cortisol, epinephrine, norepinephrine, and many other things in it. Many practitioners feel that this gives very good results for improving low cortisol. Ask your functional practitioner for specific recommendations for any glandular product, as you must use a high-quality product.

If your problem is high cortisol with anxiety or agitation, there are other things that work well. The most well-known are L-theanine and phosphatidylserine (PS). L-theanine is a very powerful amino acid. It slows your brain waves down. Normally, if you are awake and actively engaging in thought or performance, your brain waves are beta waves. These represent arousal and high thought activity. This is great during the day, but at bedtime you probably don't want a lot of beta waves. People who just can't slow down their brain have a lot of beta waves.

The slower type of brain wave are alpha waves. These are present when you finish an activity and sit down to take a break. These are predominant when you are walking on a beach. These are what you have when you first wake up or are getting tired. They represent relaxation and non-arousal. When you get tired in the evening, you are moving from beta to alpha waves. People that just can't shut down their mind in the evening are not good at moving from beta to alpha waves.

L-theanine is very good at helping you shift into alpha waves. 200–400 mg in the evening works very well if you have already turned off electronics and you are relaxing. It helps your brain shift into a more relaxed state. It will not make you sleepy, but it will lower anxiety and restlessness. L-theanine can also be used during the day, typically 100–200 mg, for anxious thoughts and agitation with difficulty focusing. It helps you calm down enough to focus on the task at hand and reduces anxiety. Green tea is a great afternoon pick-me-up. It has a small amount of caffeine in it, which helps focus, but it also naturally contains L-theanine. The L-theanine counteracts the little bit of caffeine, so you don't get amped up, jittery, or shaky. It helps you have good brain energy with calm focus.

Phosphatidylserine, or PS, is another good supplement to take in the evening if your evening cortisol is high. It is a lipoprotein that helps tell your pituitary gland to stop sending the signal to the adrenals, so then the adrenals slow down cortisol production. I often have my patients take PS around supper time to lower evening cortisol.

Another popular combination is phellodendron and magnolia bark. This is another natural way to calm down. It is similar to prescription anti-anxiety medication, but it is milder and non-addicting or sedating.

One more nutrient is worth mentioning here for cognitive support and focus. Nicotinamide adenine dinucleotide, or NAD+, is a form of vitamin B3 (niacin) that is crucial for your cells to generate energy. If you do not have enough NAD+, your cells get sluggish. Brain fog, lack of focus, processing delays, and mood swings can result. Nicotinamide riboside, or NR, is turned into NAD+ in the body. NR is available as a pill or nasal spray, but it only has a mild effect. NAD+ is available as an IV infusion or self-administered subcutaneous injection. It has become very well known for its ability to lift brain fog to enhance cognitive function. If you have chronic stress that is causing significant brain fog, look for a provider that offers NAD+ infusions and give it a try.

There are a lot of other helpful botanicals and nutrients you can take that help your entire HPA axis. Ask your functional medicine practitioner for advice for your situation. I will tell you what he or she should tell you—healing your adrenals (HPA axis) takes a long time. Do not expect that a supplement will work in a few days. When significant stress resolves, the HPA axis may take six to eighteen months to fully recover, depending on how severe and how long-standing the stress was. If you still have stress, it may only improve and may not totally normalize until the stressor goes away. This isn't a problem that can be solved with one bottle of pills.

Lastly, do not make the common mistake of thinking that just taking a few supplements a day is all you need to do to help your stress response. It is not! The next two chapters on psychological and spiritual approaches are, in my opinion, much more powerful than any supplement you can take. A supplement will help, but it cannot solve all your problems by itself. Fortunately, there are a lot of things you can work on for good mental health. Add to them a solid scriptural approach, and watch God work a *good work* in you!

Sleep

Sleep is tremendously important for stress resilience. Part of Navy Seal training is not sleeping for a week. Add to that all the unbelievable physical and psychological stress they go through, and it's just amazing that anyone makes it to the end of Hell Week. Those are some special soldiers!

Dr. Walker's book *Why We Sleep* talks about how sleep resets your brain. Your brain waves change during the different phases of sleep. They firm up and organize your thoughts from the day into permanent memories. Learning continues after you are asleep at the end of the day.[30]

Dr. Daniel Amen, a leading proponent of brain health, talks about how sleep cleans your brain overnight. Toxins and waste products of cellular metabolism build up during the day, and the brain eliminates them overnight. It's like having too many programs and windows open on your computer and then it gets sluggish. You reboot it, and it works great again! Sleep does that for your brain.[31]

Jeff Iliff gave a talk at TEDMED in 2014 on how the brain clears itself of waste. Since there are no lymphatics, your brain uses the cerebrospinal fluid (CSF) to clear waste. The CSF bathes the surface of the brain. We now know that the CSF flows along the outside of blood vessels to wash out waste. But there's a catch. It only does this during sleep! Something else happens during sleep: the brain cells shrink just a tiny bit, opening space in between cells, to increase the ability of the CSF to flush out waste. When the brain is awake and busy, it puts off the task of clearing waste. During sleep, the waste elimination can happen.[32]

One ominous finding of Dr. Iliff's is regarding one waste product, amyloid beta. This is the protein that builds up in the brain and accumulates in between the cells of the brain, and people with Alzheimer's have too much amyloid beta buildup. Amyloid beta is often removed while we sleep. But studies have shown that sleep deprivation leads to a buildup of amyloid beta in the brain, along with neuroinflammation and cognitive decline.[33] Sleep is definitely good for your brain!

What can you do to help sleep?

» Limit daytime naps to thirty minutes

» Exercise daily, but not within a few hours of bedtime

» Avoid stimulants like caffeine or nicotine in the afternoon

» Avoid blue light for several hours before bedtime (no phone, tablet, computer or television)

» Turn down the thermostat to 66–68° at night

» Run white noise in the bedroom

» Keep the bedroom dark

» Keep a regular routine in the evening

» Take a bath with Epsom salts and calming essential oils to relax

If you need to take something for sleep, there are a few things you can do. First, melatonin has been used for years for sleep. It has been shown to help with jet lag and shift-work disorder, because in those conditions, your brain isn't making melatonin at night when you are awake so you don't feel tired. Taking melatonin at bedtime for a few days in a new time zone can help your brain adjust. Please note that the dose of melatonin can be anywhere from 0.5 mg to 10 mg. Some people need higher doses, but for most, 1–3 mg is sufficient. Some people find that melatonin helps them fall asleep, but they still wake up in the middle of the night. A sustained release formulation may be needed then.

Melatonin is a bioidentical hormone so it is quite safe. Also, some recent studies of melatonin in cancer survivors have shown that at higher doses (10 mg or more), melatonin operates as an antioxidant and may reduce the risk of cancer recurrence.[34] If your natural melatonin level is low, taking it might be really good for you.

There are many other herbals often blended with melatonin in sleep supplements. These include:

» L-theanine

» GABA

» Valerian

» Lemon balm

» Passionflower

» 5-HTP

» CBD

These natural supplements typically help your brain unwind and fall asleep naturally. They don't cause sedation like medications do, but rather, they enhance relaxation so you can sleep normally. They are not addictive and do not cause morning sedation. Most of them have very few side effects. Most people can find a natural supplement that works with good sleep hygiene habits to give them seven to eight hours of sleep.

If natural supplements don't work, there are two kinds of sleep medications available over the counter: diphenhydramine and doxylamine. Most sleep medications you can get at the drugstore contain diphenhydramine. This is a sedating antihistamine and is the active ingredient in Benadryl®. Read the label to find the correct version for sleep. Most people will feel the sedative effect at a dose of 25–50 mg. The other one found in a drugstore is doxylamine and is also a sedating antihistamine.

Are these safe? Yes and no. Occasionally, they are fine, and they can work well. They do tend to have a longer duration of action, so they cause trouble waking up and you can have cognitive slowing in the morning. But even if that doesn't affect you, they aren't good for long term use. They disrupt a very important neurotransmitter in the brain: acetylcholine. Acetylcholine is vitally important for making and preserving memories. If you take this type of medication every night, you may be increasing your risk for dementia in the long term.

The next level of pills are prescription medications. These sleeping pills are a type of sedative called benzodiazepines. The most common are zolpidem, lorazepam, and alprazolam. These are addictive and cause tolerance issues as well as sleep disruptive behaviors. (I have heard a lot of stories about people sleep eating at night while on zolpidem. Quite often, it's chips, and they find the crumbs in bed the next day. Funny, but scary!) Also, recent research has linked these medications to an increased risk of dementia. Pretty much any of these meds will help you sleep, but at a high long-term price. Do everything you can to avoid having to take them.

Sex Hormones

Hormone balance is vitally important to how well you deal with stress! Ask any husband of a woman with PMS (premenstrual syndrome), and he'll roll his eyes as he complains about her moodiness during that time of her cycle. PMS is related to changes in your hormones and can dramatically decrease your stress resilience.

The first hormone important in regulating moods and your outlook on life is progesterone. This is made by the ovaries during the second half of the cycle. It drops off at the end of the twenty-eight-day cycle and then you get your period. One of the things that contributes to PMS is when the ovaries do not make enough progesterone the week before your period. Common symptoms are bloating, cramps, headaches, cravings, and irritability or depression.

Progesterone deficiency is very common in women over thirty-five. There are a lot of theories about why this is, but poor nutrition, stress, and toxins all are probably contributing factors. But fortunately, it is simple to replace progesterone. We typically use progesterone either as a pill or a cream, and if you have regular cycles, you use it from the middle of your cycle until you get your period. This works for most women with their symptoms of PMS. If you have significant trouble sleeping, the pill form of progesterone usually works much better than the cream at helping you sleep on a deeper level.

Estrogen can also contribute to stress issues. High estrogen is sometimes seen when progesterone is low. We call this estrogen dominance. Sometimes your ovaries just make too much, and sometimes it is a detoxing issue, where your liver isn't very efficient at eliminating it. High estrogen can cause symptoms similar to PMS: fluid retention, breast tenderness, bloating, and irritability. When you have this, you probably aren't going to react to stresses optimally. We treat this by adding progesterone to balance it out, as well as nutrients to increase detoxification of estrogens, such as I3C, diindolylmethane, and calcium D-glucarate. When estrogen is low, though, you usually know it! This is what happens around menopause. Your periods start spacing out, and you get hot flashes and night sweats. Your brain also usually isn't quite as sharp as it used to be. Women often report overall brain fog, trouble with memory, and lack of focus. Adding bioidentical estrogen can work wonders for these symptoms. We use estrogen as a cream, patch, or pellet. Most of us trained in integrative medicine will not use estrogen as a pill, though. When taken orally, estrogen (even bioidentical) will affect blood clotting factors and increase your risk of blood clots, heart attack, and stroke. No, thank you!

One of the most powerful hormones for mood and mental vitality is testosterone. One of the hallmarks of low testosterone in men is fatigue and irritability. These guys can feel like they are stuck on the couch with no motivation to do anything and no zest for life. They often get irritable and angry. Women also complain of physical and mental fatigue when their testosterone is low. They just aren't motivated to get out there and do anything.

Testosterone has three main functions:

1. **Sex.** Yes, you have a better sex drive when your testosterone is good! We all know that in our upper teens to our twenties, most of us have a healthy sex drive. While it can get you into trouble, it is how we were designed to feel. Most couples remember what it felt like to get married and then enjoy a very good sex life, at least for a while. Until stress and kids come into the picture, that is! Testosterone not only gives you sexual thoughts and drive; it also enhances the sexual response. You have more blood flow to the genital region and better nerve response, so it just feels good. Men get better erections. Women are more able to reach orgasm. It is possible to have good sex without optimal testosterone levels, but when your hormone levels are normal, it will be a bigger part of your relationship and give you more joy.

2. **Muscle mass.** Testosterone is very important to building muscle. Without good levels, you may work out frequently, but you won't be able to improve your performance, and you may not feel as strong as you should. You may not be able to gain muscle with your workouts, and it may take you awhile to recover from a hard workout.

3. **Brain health.** Many people are unaware of testosterone's effect on the brain. Without testosterone, most people are unmotivated,

poorly focused, and irritable. They just don't want to do much of anything, and their moods are poor. Depression, anxiety, and irritability are common. Combine stressful events in life with low testosterone, and you won't handle it as well as you should.

Testosterone is sometimes used as a cream but can also be used as an injection or as pellets. Creams and other topical forms of testosterone have only a mild effect, and thus are usually insufficient in men. Most men in my practice are on injections or pellets, and they feel great. Women do sometimes use testosterone as a cream, but it only has a mild effect on boosting moods and brain function. Quite often women also prefer pellet therapy. Pellets are bioidentical hormone made into a small pellet the size of a grain of rice. They are inserted under the skin in a quick office procedure every three to four months and provide a nice, steady level of testosterone in your system. Most people feel more energy, focus, and better moods within one to two weeks of pellet placement. Injections are also another option. This also gives your brain nice levels of testosterone for a good brain-boosting effect. However, giving yourself injections once or twice a week is a lot of work and somewhat painful, so it's not a popular choice.

Those of us who specialize in bioidentical hormone replacement therapy (BHRT) can tell you many stories of patients who are doing amazingly well with this treatment. Many of my patients can feel a big difference in their overall energy, their moods, their motivation, and their overall stress resilience when they are on BHRT.

Some have questioned the use of BHRT, claiming it's not natural. The argument is that if hormone levels go down in middle age, it must be part of God's plan, so we should leave it that way. People also wonder if BHRT is somehow masking the real issue. However, consider that life expectancy now is about thirty years after menopause. We are living longer and healthier lives, well after our natural youthful hormone levels drop. I firmly believe that in a perfect world, the healthy levels of hormones that occur in the reproductive years would continue indefinitely. But we live in a fallen world, and our hormone levels decline.

There is abundant evidence that many diseases of aging are accelerated by the drop in hormones that occurs in middle age. In fact, estrogen, progesterone, and testosterone all have research showing they reduce the risk of heart disease, both for men[35] and women.[36] Furthermore, dementia[37] and osteoporosis[38] are reduced when BHRT is used. Lastly, believe it or not, there is emerging data that indicates several types of cancer occur less often in women who are put on BHRT.[39]

Maintaining youthful levels of hormones into our senior years is associated with less diseases of aging. We are preserving God's design for the function of our bodies, and we feel better as a result. When we feel better physically and emotionally, stress has much less of an effect on us. That's a win all around.

Thyroid

Thyroid health is important to address while you work on other areas affected by stress. As we briefly looked at earlier, stress suppresses the conversion of fT4 to fT3. Here is the reaction, with a list of all the nutrients needed for the conversion.

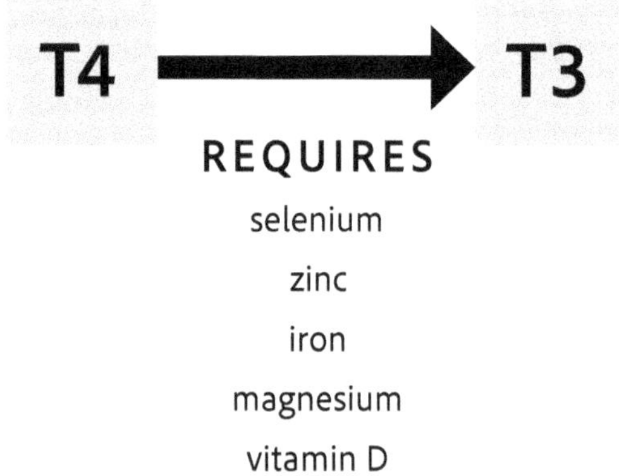

If you do not have all these nutrients in adequate amounts, you will not convert as much fT4 to fT3 and therefore, your cellular metabolism will drop. Remember, the thyroid hormone is like gasoline to the engine of the cell. When you have enough thyroid hormone and it goes into the cell, the cell works efficiently. Without enough thyroid hormone, the cellular engine slows down.

If your TSH is over 5, you need to take thyroid hormone. Although many probably do not like to take prescription medication, I will assure you that thyroid hormone is virtually side-effect free when taken correctly and as directed by a physician, and many types are totally bioidentical. The porcine thyroid hormones, such as Armour® and NP Thyroid®, are not bioidentical (they come from pigs), but interestingly, they often work better for symptom relief.[40] However, levothyroxine works well most of the time and is bioidentical. If you have symptoms of hypothyroidism and an elevated TSH level, please trust your physician and start thyroid hormone. You will feel better, which will help you with stress, sleep, and other physical issues. You may have more energy, have more regular bowel movements, and may lose weight. Wouldn't that be nice?

If your TSH isn't that high, you may only need supplements. Most good supplement companies have a thyroid supporting product that includes a combination of several of these ingredients:

- » Vitamin A
- » Vitamin C
- » Vitamin E
- » Selenium
- » Tyrosine
- » Zinc
- » Iodine
- » Guggul

A word about iodine: Many people mistakenly think that when it comes to iodine, more is better. There have been physicians who have advocated for high dose iodine therapy, but this is not recommended. While the US RDA for iodine is 150 mcg, most people only need about 150–1000 mcg per day, or up to 1 mg per day. Doses above 5–10 mg taken on a long-term basis may suppress your thyroid function.[41] This is controversial, and some doctors routinely use iodine at 25–50 mg per day, but there isn't good research showing that this is necessary. The concern is that high doses of iodine can cause hyperthyroidism, or an overstimulation of the thyroid gland. It's not common, but don't take high dose iodine on your own. Talk to your provider. Urine testing is available to check your level of iodine and to guide your dosing, so let your provider guide you. Most supplements will provide 150–300 mcg iodine, which is just fine for thyroid support.

If you have hypothyroidism, you should be aware that raw cruciferous vegetables and soy-based foods are something you shouldn't eat every day. Soy-based food, which include soy milk, tofu, tempeh, and edamame, contain an isoflavone called genistein which can suppress thyroid hormone production.[42] This doesn't mean you can't ever eat soy-based foods, but just don't make a habit of eating them every day. The other food group to limit is cruciferous vegetables such as broccoli, cauliflower, Brussels sprouts, and cabbage. They contain isothiocyanates which also can mildly suppress thyroid hormone production.[43]

What we don't know, however, is how much of an effect these foods have on your thyroid. There is evidence that cooking both soy and cruciferous vegetables diminishes the effect on the thyroid, but of course, cooking crucifers lessens their nutritional value. The other consideration is that if you are on thyroid medication, eating these foods won't affect you as much, because you are taking your thyroid hormone in a pill and are not totally dependent on your thyroid to make its own. In general, just try to avoid eating a lot of these foods. If you keep your consumption reasonable and consistent, you can eat them.

Gut Health

The relationship between gut health and our stress response is under appreciated. However, the gut-brain connection has been talked about much more often in the past decade. For years, we have observed that there is an association between gastrointestinal disorders, autoimmune disorders, and mental health issues. Autoimmune disease is largely connected to leaky gut and gut inflammation.[44] It turns out that anything that affects the brain, like stress, can affect the gut and vice versa.

What is the gut-brain connection? There are a number of connections. The first is that about 90 percent of your serotonin is produced in the intestinal cells.[45] Serotonin is the neurotransmitter that is crucial for a good mood. When it is depleted, depression and anxiety occur. Although antidepressants that support serotonin in the brain are often helpful, you can't ignore a common underlying reason: poor gut health sending signals to the brain.

As explained in earlier chapters, the microbiome is the unique makeup of all the bacteria in your intestinal tract. Our microbiome is affected by the food we eat, our stress, chemicals we are exposed to, and medications, in particular, antibiotics. When our microbiome is unhealthy, our brains often feel it. There was an interesting study done that shows an important way the gut and brain are connected. Mice were engineered to have a lack in normal gut bacteria. They showed a significant decrease in fear extinction learning. That mean that a normal mouse learns after a while that a particular fear is not reasonable, and over time, the fear disappears. The abnormal mice showed a significantly reduced ability to learn that a threatening danger was no longer present. In other words, they continued to act out of anxiety and fear.[46] Why did this happen? The microglia, which are immune cells in the brain, did not get the right signals from the gut bacteria. Instead of doing their normal function of remodeling neurons, they failed. Bacteria in the gut will send signals to the brain and will change your brain. Wow!

If your gut is healthy, your brain will be better equipped to respond to stressful situations with grace and resilience. But the opposite is also true: if you eat junk food and have an inflamed, leaky gut, your brain just won't be able to handle stress. Small things will get you angry or depressed, making the battle ten times harder. Have you ever gone to a conference or to a fancy meal somewhere that included a lot of healthy whole foods? One of the benefits of being in anti-aging medicine is that conference meals are usually extremely healthy. (When I was in family medicine, sandwiches and cookies were common.) When you eat a healthy salad with some protein and fruit for lunch, how do you feel? Compare that to if you ate a fast-food hamburger and fries. When you eat real food in normal portions, you feel energized, as you should. But eating a fast-food meal doesn't usually give you much energy. Your GI tract has to work hard to process all that fake food.

There is a huge correlation between how much real, whole food you eat and how healthy your brain is. Sugar, white flour, preservatives, and unhealthy fats can weigh your brain down. Eat meat (grass-fed beef, free-range chicken, and wild-caught fish are best), organic eggs, beans, brown rice, quinoa, nuts, and as many fruits and vegetables as you can. Avoid sugar, starchy foods, alcohol, beverages other than water, tea, and coffee, or anything else fake and processed. You will feel better. And if you feel better physically and/or mentally, you are much better equipped to adapt to stress. You will see situations clearly and will be able to respond calmly and with wisdom, instead of letting emotions rule the day. "Let food be thy medicine, and let medicine be thy food" is widely attributed to Hippocrates.[47] Although those exact words do not appear in the surviving Hippocratic Corpus, the concept has always been true and always will be. Eat healthy, real food, and your body will do what it is capable of.

But if your gut is not healthy, you need to fix it. The first thing to do is get tested with a stool test and test for food sensitivities, like we discussed in the previous chapter. That way you know exactly how to adjust your diet. There are also supplements that are used for various digestive issues.

Digestive enzymes are very useful for indigestion, heartburn, or reflux. A good enzyme will have protease, lipase, cellulase, amylase, and other ingredients to digest all types of food. You take them with a meal, and they help your stomach pre-digest the food.

Supplements to heal leaky gut can be pills or powders, and they include ingredients such as:

> » L-glutamine
>
> » Deglycyrrhized Licorice Root Extract

- » N-acetyl-D-glucosamine

- » Aloe vera

- » Okra

- » Slippery elm bark

- » Marshmallow root

- » Ginger

- » Colostrum or SBI (serum bovine immunoglobulins)

Talk to your provider about how long you should take them.

Probiotics are crucial if you have any dysbiosis. Probiotics reinoculate the gut with beneficial strains of bacteria. There are a wide variety of probiotics out there, and unfortunately, many are of poor quality and don't have very many bacteria in them. You want a product with a blend of different bacterial strains in it, and you want at least 10 billion bacteria per capsule, if not higher. Do not buy probiotics from a large chain store. Shop at a reputable health food store or ask your provider for a recommendation.

CHAPTER 6

Psychological Strategies for Healing

In some respects, what we need to talk about now is a lot harder than the strictly medical stuff. It's one thing to change your diet and take supplements. Some of us love to tackle a detailed plan and follow it to the letter. Some of my patients come in with a big bag of supplements because they have done hours of research into their symptoms and have tried to treat themselves. I admire their effort! But sometimes the solution needs to go much deeper than taking pills. We need to do some deep self-assessment, down where it hurts, and untangle some of the messes in our mind. I like to say it's like after the cat played with the ball of yarn all over the living room. Untangling that mess and slowly rewinding it takes time and a lot of effort, and it often isn't any fun at all.

I'm good at taking my supplements. I am disciplined, like a lot of doctors are. If I need zinc, by golly, I'm going to take it every day. Curcumin with ginger for inflammation? Done. Fish oil? Easy. I rarely forget to take my supplements. But it's been about two weeks since I've been able to work on this book. Gosh darn it, I was totally in the zone a few weeks ago, writing every day, thinking how well I was doing with the stress in my life. Then it all came to a screeching halt because of a major stressor. This was much greater than any adrenal supplement would help. (God often has to knock us down a few notches when we think we have it all figured out. Have you ever noticed that?)

Our family had a particularly stressful weekend. Daniel was especially irritable and noticeably struggling for days. Everything got him upset, he needed our attention every few minutes, and he was being destructive with his electronic devices. *All day long.* On Sunday, he was reaching out trying to hit me by eight-thirty in the morning. I was frazzled to the core. When we experience days like this, my husband and I manage as best we can and try not to take out our frustration on each other.

Guess what happened? You got it—my husband and I got mad at each other over something really dumb. I think most couples have that one issue they disagree about. For some it's the toothpaste tube, for some it's laundry or dishes, but for us it's about me not waking him up when I wake up first.

I am usually the early bird, up at dawn. My husband is a night owl. And then let's also acknowledge the years and years we spent sleep deprived from caring for Daniel in the middle of the night. We still experience PTSD symptoms from those hard, sleepless years. The result is that now my husband often struggles to sleep at night, and he just doesn't wake up early easily.

On Sunday morning, I was up dealing with an irritable autistic teenager, and my husband was sleeping. I thought he had been up with Daniel during the night, and I thought I was being nice to let him sleep. I was feeling pretty good about myself. Daniel and I got ready and were going to go to church. But my husband got up five minutes before we left and was mad at me for not waking him. We were now late to church, and I got mad in return. I'm sure you can imagine the conversation, both the spoken words and the unspoken:

Gretchen: "I thought you were up with Daniel last night, so I let you sleep." *(Aren't I great?)*

Hubby: "No, I wasn't. Why didn't you wake me up?" *(I can't believe you didn't let me help you!)*

Gretchen: "I was handling it fine." *(You are a grown man—why can't you wake yourself up?)*

Hubby: "No, you weren't handling it!" *(She doesn't want my help, and she clearly doesn't respect me at all!)*

See how quickly this turns into a full-fledged argument? I readily admit that I didn't handle it well, and I sulked for a few days. It took me awhile to really see that my bravado and supposed strength were not only foolish but disrespectful to myself and my husband. My behavior was also full of pride.

Here's a basic principle we too often forget—God gives us others to help us! As women, we are so often deceived into thinking we must do it all and somehow manage, but we don't let ourselves ask for help. This is the sin of pride. John writes, "For all that is in the world—the lust of the flesh, the lust of the eyes, and the pride of life—is not of the Father but is of the world" (1 John 2:16). We read in the Proverbs, "By pride comes nothing but strife, but with the well-advised is wisdom" (Proverbs 13:10) and, "In the mouth of a fool is a rod of pride, but the lips of the wise will preserve them" (Proverbs 14:3).

After a few days of walking on eggshells in our house, I finally realized that I was frustrated with the challenges of parenting a child with special needs, and I was indulging in self-pity for something I brought on by my choice to not ask for help. How stupid is that? But I bet you have done the same thing at some point. I had to ask for forgiveness, and we worked through the situation. I'm now much better at asking for help, and he doesn't need me to wake him up anymore. Win-win!

Before we get into specific psychological strategies for dealing with stressful situations, remember that the basic formula for dealing with stress is a four-step approach:

1. Separate what you can control from what you can't.

2. Do what you can. Choose a good attitude and peace. (Do *your* part.)

3. Ask for help (for the *other* part).

4. Make a habit of self-nurture.

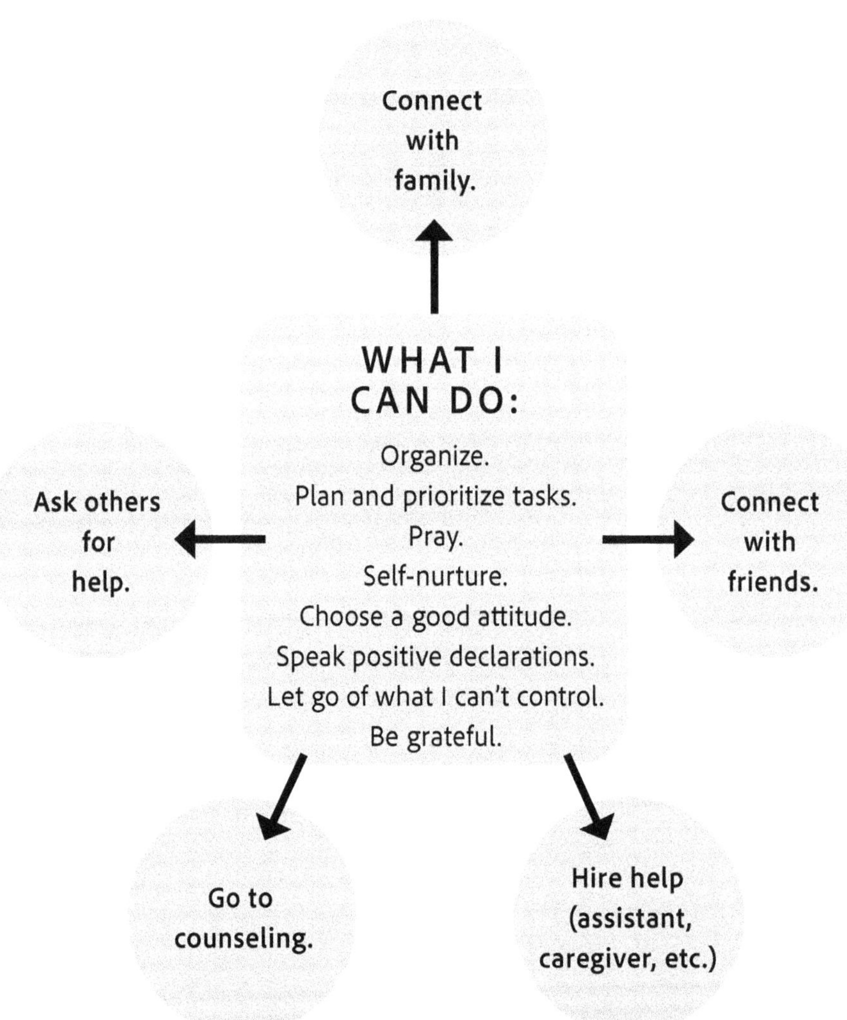

CREATE A MIND MAP.

1. Separate what you can control from what you can't

The first thing you need to do is to separate what you can control from what you can't. This is not always easy and not always obvious. When you are afraid, disappointed, or frustrated, your emotions often interfere with clear, rational thought.

In my example of the challenging weekend we experienced with Daniel, I couldn't change the fact that everything was frustrating to him. I couldn't make him stop crying. I couldn't restrain him from hitting. But what I could do was stand several feet away. I could keep him out of striking distance of the computer, iPad, and headphones. I could take him for a drive in the car as a change in scenery. I could try to make silly voices with his stuffed animals to make him laugh. Did I? *Nope.* I was a basket case, filled with frustration and on the verge of crying. My emotions totally clouded my ability to think rationally.

If you need to write ideas down, do it. I admit I'm middle-aged, and I grew up in the era before laptops. I somehow managed to get through school, college, and medical school with notebooks and pens. I still take notes at conferences in a notebook. Research shows that the physical act of writing things down helps your brain process the information. Make a list of the things you can and can't control, and it will become much more clear to you.

2. Do what you can. Choose a good attitude and peace.

When you see clearly what you can control, make a plan and act on it. Choose to have a good attitude, no matter what you might feel. Emotions are real and they can be intense, but God doesn't want us to act only based on emotions. He expects us to be mature Christians and to discern the right path, using our faith, even when we don't feel like it. Paul tells us, "Brethren, I do not count myself to have apprehended; but one thing I do, forgetting those things which are behind and reaching forward to those things which are ahead, I press toward the goal for the prize of the upward call of God in Christ Jesus. Therefore let us, as many as are mature, have this mind" (Philippians 3:13–15).

"Behind" means something in the past or behind you in time. We are called to move forward and toward better things, not allowing emotions to move with us into the future. They are what they are and may be totally justified, but we have the choice whether we allow them to cling to us in the future or if we leave them at the altar.

The "upward call" or "high calling" in verse 14 means a summons or an invitation to a heavenly or higher place. This means we are expected to choose a better response instead of just succumbing to earthly emotions. In verse 15, we see that if we do so, we are mature in our faith.

Paul later writes, "And now, dear brothers and sisters, one final thing. Fix your thoughts on what is true, and honorable, and right, and pure, and lovely, and admirable. Think about things that are excellent and worth of praise. Keep putting into practice all you learned and receive from me—everything you heard from me and saw me doing. Then the God of peace will be with you." (Philippians 4:8–9 NLT). I love this version. "Fix your thoughts" makes it clear it is an intentional act. Do not let yourself dwell in past emotion, but instead control your thoughts. Keep practicing this habit and you will be filled with peace. Those painful emotions will fade much more quickly when they are replaced with positive, faith-filled thoughts. The choice of what we think about is always totally up to us.

In my case with Daniel, I did do what I could physically. I removed myself and any electronics out of Daniel's reach, and we still got of the house and went to church. I totally failed with the emotional aspect. I stewed in anger and let my feelings control my attitude for days. Romans 8:6 says, "For to be carnally minded is death, but to be spiritually minded is life and peace." If you live in the emotions of the flesh, you will pay the price and be stressed and unwell. The fruit of strife is rotten and destructive to your soul. Leave it behind and embrace life-giving, peaceful thoughts!

3. Ask for help.

This is difficult for many of us, especially if we have had a lot of struggles in life. If you grew up in a not-so-good home, if you had to put yourself through school, or if you are a single parent, then you have had to work hard to get where you are. This is a great strength, but your weakness may be that you are not good at asking for help. Some of us are incredibly good at taking care of everyone else but we are resistant to offers of help. We can be blind to the fact that we are an emotional mess and need help.

God gives us others because we are stronger together. Ecclesiastes tells us, "Two are better than one, because they have a good reward for their labor. For if they fall, one will lift up his companion. But woe to him who is alone when he falls, for he has no one to help him up. Again, if two lie down together, they will keep warm; but how can one be warm alone? Though one may be overpowered by another, two can withstand him. And a threefold cord is not quickly broken" (Ecclesiastes 4:9–12).

Surround yourself with good friends and invest in your relationships with others. Connect with them and help others any way you can. I taught my children that you should always accept extra shifts at work and always offer to help others, whether it is moving on a Saturday or giving someone a ride. When you give of yourself when you can, you will find out that others will be glad to help you out when it's your turn to need help. You can call it karma, but I call it "The Law of Sowing and Reaping." Sow into others with a generous spirit and you will reap later when you need help.

Some of us find it hard to accept gifts. Whether it's a compliment we brush off or an offer of help we decline, we won't allow others to help. This blocks two blessings: your blessing in receiving the gift and the other person's blessing of giving. When you give to someone, how do you feel? One year, we gave a gift of a few hundred dollars to our church to buy Christmas trees for those who couldn't afford them. This was above and beyond our normal tithes and offering, and I can't tell you how good it felt to know that we blessed several families with the joy of a Christmas tree! The feeling of joy and satisfaction that results from giving is a great blessing that you just can't explain unless you experience it.

When you decline a gift, whether it is money, time, or a physical gift, you are stealing the blessing the giver would have experienced. When you graciously accept help, you are bringing life into your own circumstances but are also unleashing blessing upon the giver. Giving leads us to give more, which leads others to give more, and that's how God operates. God is love and He gives to us all the time, while we give back to Him and to others. Don't be guilty of blocking blessings. Receive gifts graciously and allow others to help you when you need it. You will then give it forward to someone else when you can.

I have a patient I will call Anna, who is such a joy to me and my staff. Every time she comes in, she is so full of energy and joy that she completely brightens up the office. I hate to even charge her for her visits because she gives so much to us spiritually. She comes with a small gift for myself and my front office staff, usually pens or small pads of paper. Because it is a small gift, we can accept it and we are so thankful. When I use that silver pen with pink flowers on it, I always think of Anna, and my spirit is filled with appreciation. I know Anna enjoys giving because she does it everywhere she goes. God expects us to live in community with others—in our family, in our church, and in our world. Together, we are strong.

4. Make a habit of self-nurture.

I tell my patients all the time, especially women, that we absolutely must take time to self-nurture. You know how the flight attendant on every flight tells you to put on your own oxygen mask first before assisting the person next to you? Do you know why that is? It only takes a few seconds at altitude for you to pass out without oxygen. In those precious few seconds, you are helping yourself stay conscious so that you are able to help someone else. Similarly, when you are psychologically not conscious of your situation or emotions, you are essentially useless to everyone else.

When you aren't taking care of yourself, you will not be effective in what you are trying to do. Poor emotional health causes inattention, irritability, and a lack of clear thinking. This makes your work much more difficult and error prone.

Have you ever had to go to work right after you had an argument with a loved one? Or gotten reprimanded by a supervisor in the middle of the day in front of others? Think about how you felt emotionally in that moment. When you had to resume your work duties, how well did you do? I would guess poorly. You probably weren't focused, instead thinking about the negative situation and trying to plan out your next steps. You may have been a little snippy with a coworker. The ball of yarn of your emotions was totally unwound all over the place and you just couldn't think straight.

Self-nurture involves many strategies. Start thinking about what truly gives you peace and what brings you joy. I have a few hobbies that do that. I also have learned that sometimes what I really need when I come home in the evening is to take a twenty-minute hot bath with essential oils. Ask your spouse for a massage—sometimes, a ten-minute foot rub is all you need. Go for a walk outside—listen to the birds and notice the squirrels or the other people walking their dogs. Carve out thirty minutes to read a good fiction book. Whatever brings you calm and happiness is crucial to your overall health.

I encourage you to start a journal right now. Later in this chapter we will talk more about journaling, but take time right now to write down activities that soothe you or give you joy. Make this personal and easily applicable to your life. If you learn nothing else from this book, adding self-nurture regularly to your schedule will help immensely. Enjoy it without feeling guilty at all. You deserve it!

Let's now look at different ways of dealing with negative thoughts and emotions. We'll discuss how to process them, how to examine them for the good and the bad, and how to purposely choose the most productive path through them. Our journey through stress reduction psychology starts now.

Meditation

Meditation used to be a word that made me nervous. A few decades ago, it was really not cool for a Christian to talk about meditating. I was told that meditation was Eastern religion and not something a good Christian should do. Some people still don't quite understand what meditation is, so they shy away from it. However, meditation is all throughout Scripture.

We are commanded to meditate! It simply means to contemplate, consider, and deeply think about something. We are supposed to meditate on God, because our natural tendency is to think about the things and people we see and interact with, not the invisible God. The only way to keep focused on God through our day is to, in a sense, force ourselves to think about him. It's like putting on a pair of filtered sunglasses. You still see everything, but if you filter out the unimportant things and look through a God filter, you see things differently.

Psalm 4:4 says, "Be angry, and do not sin. Meditate within your heart on your bed, and be still." And Psalm 77:1–12 tells us, "I cried out to God with my voice—To God with my voice; And He gave ear to me. In the day of my trouble I sought the Lord; My hand was stretched out in the night without ceasing; My soul refused to be comforted. I remembered God, and was troubled; I complained, and my spirit was overwhelmed . . . I call to remembrance my song in the night; I meditate within my heart, And my spirit makes diligent search . . . I will remember the works of the LORD . . . I will also meditate on all Your work and talk of Your deeds."

Paul writes in his letter to the Philippians, "Finally brethren, whatever things are true, whatever things are noble, whatever things are just, whatever things are pure, whatever things are lovely, whatever things are of good report . . . meditate on these things" (Philippians 4:8).

In the first verse, the psalmist addresses anger. Anger itself is an emotion we all experience and is not sinful. But what you do with it makes all the difference. I find it interesting the psalmist says to be still while you meditate. Sit down, put the phone away, turn off the television, and just be still. Your anger will be diffused the longer you are still. Sometimes, when I am upset and frantic, one of my older sons will say to me, "Mom, calm down!" He is right, of course, so when he gives me that mild verbal rebuke, I grudgingly realize that I do need to slow down and relax. Likewise, when you have a child who is upset, what do you do? You try to comfort them by getting them to calm down. Being still is a great way to bring peace.

In Psalm 77, David is in deep trouble and in emotional anguish. He reached out to God "in the night without ceasing." He prayed for a long time without relief and felt hopeless, and he was even complaining! If even the mighty David felt hopeless and complained loudly, the same will happen to all of us. But here's the thing: he didn't stay there. He purposely remembered a song, he intentionally meditated on God, and he made himself remember the works of God. He felt those negative emotions so strongly that he almost gave up. But he didn't.

We always have a choice in how we respond. The very first thing we need to do is recognize we are in a pit of negativity. It may or may not be your fault at all. When someone reminds you to chill out, you need to wake up and see how your attitude is affecting you. No matter why you're in that mud pit of despair, you totally have a choice about how you're going to respond.

Many people stay mired in anger, frustration, and depression. They lash out at anyone around them for no reason. They are probably mad at themselves but unwilling to admit it. They are too proud to ask God or anyone else for help and they take it out on everyone else, further alienating themselves. This is only a recipe for further destruction. You may start at a very shallow level, but, with further poor choices of how to respond, you dig yourself deeper until you are depressed, alone, and unsuccessful in life.

Meditation acts like a stop sign. When the storm winds blow, you will feel battered, hurt, and exhausted. You need to stop. Be still. *Rest.* This is exactly what God is waiting for you to do. Once you do, you can slowly reverse the situation. Meditation is often used in Eastern religious traditions, but it is very compatible with Christianity, so do not be afraid.

How do we meditate? To meditate means to engage in thought and contemplation. I was taught years ago as a new Christian to make meditation part of my daily prayer time, with worship, praise, repentance, focused prayers for self, prayers for others, reading scripture, and a time of silent reflection. I was taught right away that you have to basically shut up and listen. In my Pentecostal church, people prayed a lot and prayed loud! Many people thought prayer meant constant loud chatter to God. I had to learn to be quiet and spend time just listening. It's amazing how often

God is trying to talk to you, but you keep yammering away in prayer and miss what He's trying to tell you.

Meditation does not have to be only within prayer time, though. There are many ways to meditate, but most people recommend you sit comfortably in a chair and start with ten minutes of doing nothing. That's right—*nothing*. Sit with your feet flat on the floor and rest your hands comfortably. Set your timer and then close your eyes.

When you are learning to meditate, simply make observations. What different sounds do you hear? Do you feel air moving in the room? Do you smell anything? How does your body feel in the chair? Consider what all five senses are telling you. Take slow comfortable breaths. When thoughts start to occupy your mind (*which they will*), simply observe them and then let them go. Make room for the next thought. Most of us don't use all our senses enough. I love to walk my dog on a wooded path by a nearby lake. The smell, the crunch of leaves underfoot, the sound of a distant boat or a bird, and the different appearance of the lake every day are beautiful. A good way to learn how to meditate it to sit outside or near an open window.

Listen to all the different sounds, both inside and outside. Can you hear different bird sounds? Do you hear any traffic? Frogs? The buzzing of a bee? The fan of your HVAC system? Do you smell anything? Feel how the floor feels under your feet. Feel how relaxed your arms and hands are. Feel the world around you without using your eyesight. Be present in the moment and let thoughts come and go, but do not dwell on anything. When your timer goes off, open your eyes and sit for another minute. Notice how relaxed your muscles are. Feel how calm your spirit is.

Most beginners find it challenging to keep thoughts from taking over their thinking, but with time, you will find it easier to let them move on. You will simply be in the present, not doing anything, not thinking anything in particular, but just being. This is very powerful. We spend most of our waking time thinking things or doing things. Several generations ago, folks used to sit on the front porch in the evening and would visit with neighbors. They might sit out there for hours. Have you ever been on vacation with family and done just that? Beautiful, right?

With meditation, you learn to separate from your emotions over your situation. You can be more objective and make rational choices about how to respond. This is the first step in overcoming. In Alcoholics Anonymous, you learn to acknowledge your problem first and own it. Then you can move forward in the right direction. Meditation helps us calm down and define our problem. Then and only then can we move forward climbing out of our mud pit to get victory.

Prayer

You could fill an entire library with all the books that have been written on prayer. I am not going to pretend to be an expert. I have never been to seminary, and I haven't studied the Bible in Hebrew and Greek. But you know what? I know what prayer is and how powerful it is. So do you! Prayer is between you and God. Whether you have been a Christian for fifty years or are still trying to figure out if this Jesus thing is for you, you can pray.

As Christians, we are guilty of making prayer way more complicated than it needs to be. As a young adult and new believer in a charismatic church, I remember going to the prayer room before Sunday evening service. The prayer room was filled with people praying loudly, sometimes even in tongues. I thought that to really pray, you had to be intense, loud, and emotional. I thought God didn't really pay much attention to us quiet praying folks. I prayed quietly, but I felt guilty, like I just wasn't quite as spiritual as I should be.

But then I got wise counsel from an older woman in church who had lived for God all her life. She taught me that prayer is just you and God talking, like he's sitting right next to you as your friend. She was short in stature and always prayed very quietly, but she was one of the most powerful women I have ever met. I realized that when you talk to your best friend, you don't have to yell. After all, if you're in a restaurant with your spouse, you say things to each other in a relatively quiet voice (especially the inside jokes). You don't shout, "Honey, you look so amazing tonight! I love you! You are incredible!" Nope. Those things aren't really for everyone else to hear. It's for your lover to hear.

I've been to a lot of different churches since then. In some churches, there is a time for shouting or praising God loudly. But prayer can be still and intimate. You won't ever overcome your stress and grow from it without prayer. Every stress God puts you through is to refine your character or to teach you a lesson. Let God work through it. Ultimately, you can become stronger so you can later minister to someone else.

Pray every day. Make time when you can be alone with God. (You probably won't just happen to find time. You'll have to make time for prayer.) Talk to Him like you're talking to a friend or your dad. Give Him your stresses and confess your emotions. When you submit it all to Him, He can start the healing process. Repent anything you've done to make it worse or even for not seeking His help soon enough. Give up control. Submit yourself to His will and then watch Him start to work on you. You are on the right path, moving in the right direction. Even if you have a long way to go, you're making progress.

I love to call God one of his Hebrew names Jehovah Shalom, or God of Peace. When I am stressed, I will whisper this seven times to relax. Say "Jehovah Shalom" on your breath in, then "the Lord is my peace" on your breath out. Repeat a total of seven times. This has never failed to relax me. There is power is speaking the name of God.

Nothing Time

As I mentioned in an earlier chapter, when I was growing up, I kept a diary. I would be faithful for a few weeks to write down a lot of things, but then I would slack off. Many days, I would only write, "Today was a nothing day." That is about the only thing I remember from my diaries, except for working hard to hide it from my sister!

As an adult and a parent, do you ever crave *nothing days*? I sure do! The empty time that was so unpleasant as a child is so wonderful now, because now we don't have enough of it. We need to first learn to appreciate unscheduled time as the beautiful gift it is, and then we need to schedule more of it. It is like a blank canvas that is waiting for us to paint a beautiful painting on. An extension of meditation is making time for doing absolutely nothing. Sometimes we just need to stop. We are running on a hamster wheel, exhausted, but not really getting anywhere.

When I was growing up, I loved to go camping. I loved going on hikes and finding a waterfall or a scenic overlook. We would stop and sit for a while, doing nothing but enjoying nature. We also spent a lot of time sitting around a campfire, talking and being together. I spent a lot of time just gazing into the campfire, lost deep in thought, being one with nature and the sights and smells all around me. There were no cell phones back then and certainly no television out in the woods. I didn't even like it when someone had a radio on . . . it was too "normal" for the beauty of nature.

My parents sold the house we all grew up in several years ago to buy a condo that was only one story and much easier to take care of. The one thing I really miss from that house, though, was the front porch swing. Dad had a two-person porch swing, and he loved to sit out and drink his coffee in the morning or relax in the evening. It was in a great family neighborhood where lots of folks walked around the block, especially after dinner. Dad would always greet them with a wave and *"Evening!"* The neighbors next door had two daughters who grew up coming over to hang out with him on the porch swing, like a grandfather. I loved sitting out there with him when I came home to visit. This is not something a lot of us do now—maybe because we don't build front porches on our McMansions, or maybe because no one has any unscheduled time to simply sit awhile in the evenings. I sure miss that.

Sitting on a porch swing may or may not be something you can do where you live, but you can unschedule some of your time. You don't have to have things to do in the evenings. Learn to say no to kids' activities and extra commitments. You don't have to be doing something every waking moment. Watching something on television with your spouse can be relaxing. But turning off the television and having a cup of tea can be even more relaxing. Go for a walk. Sit out on the porch after sunset and listen to the night. Can I say this again? *Turn off the television!* It's not worth your time. Don't even get me started on the news. Even when the news is correct, it's full of fear and will only increase your stress. It's okay to turn it off.

You probably won't just find time to relax. You must dedicate time, purposely and intentionally. Schedule it in your day, even if it's only fifteen minutes. Nothing time is a beautiful thing.

Journaling

Journaling is very therapeutic. I go through phases in my Christian walk when I am really good at bringing my journal to church, taking notes, and adding to it during the week. I'll do well for a month or two, then I forget. Suddenly it will be months later, and I realize I need to start journaling again.

Journaling can be many different things. It is totally up to you how you practice this. Journaling what you do each day may not have a lot of value, but when you put time and effort into writing how you're doing emotionally and spiritually, you can grow by leaps and bounds. It also can have a therapeutic effect, providing a detox on paper. If you are struggling with negative emotions, writing them all down can make you feel better, just like having a good crying session.

Journaling has a spiritual dimension to it as well. Anytime I get insight into a scripture or hear something impactful from a sermon, I like to write it down in my journal. Then I can read it again, and over time, it gets burned into my mind. About a year ago in my journal I wrote about a message I heard called "The Movie in My Mind." It was about Mary and Martha and how Martha totally had a script in her mind about how her day was going to go. Then, unexpectedly, Jesus showed up. Her plans completely went out the window. She got herself all stressed out with the work of serving a guest, and she totally missed what God wanted her to do. This is a message I could read every week and it will never grow old.

When you journal, take a few minutes to be still and listen for God. While He rarely talks to any of us in an audible voice, He will bring thoughts to your mind. If He leads you to look up Scripture, do it. Sometimes it's just a word that comes to me, and then I use the concordance in the back of my Bible to look up that word. It's amazing how God will speak to you through His Word. It is powerful, timely and always fresh for your circumstances. When God speaks to you, write it down in your journal. I also recommend that once every few months you take time on a Saturday to read your journal entries. Quite often I am refreshed and encouraged again by something I wrote down months ago but haven't kept front and center in my mind.

When you journal, I encourage you to put all your emotions and thoughts on the paper. Then take time to dig deep into why you feel the way you do, even if you discover that you have contributed to your stress by your choices. Challenge yourself to write down actionable things you can do to reduce your stress. Add scriptures that are particularly meaningful to you right now. Write down how they apply to you and what you are going to do about it.

Research studies have shown that journaling helps symptoms of depression and anxiety.[48] It can be fun, too! Buy yourself a nice journal and set of pens at your local bookstore. Let your inner child out and have fun with it! Spend several minutes each day simply writing. Don't try to edit or make it all sound just right. Let it be stream of consciousness at first. After a while, you can think deeply as you write, but at first, just get started. For you artists out there, feel free to sketch or doodle. Sometimes God shows you an image and when you get it on paper, He leads you to deeper understanding.

One more use for journaling is to document your dreams and goals. After all, once you conquer your stress response and you are living in the Spirit, you should be aiming for your life goals. Having positive direction and seeing progress can be powerfully motivating in all areas of life and can help you be more stress resilient.

I challenge you to set ten goals for yourself for the next year or so. Many of us do this in January, but no matter what month it is, do it. Get another journal or separate pages just for this.

TEN GOALS

1.
2.
3.
4.
5.
6.
7.
8.
9.
10.

Your goals can be related to your occupation, your ministry, your health or your family. Once you write down the goal, for example, to finish your college degree, draw or somehow photoshop a picture of you accomplishing that goal, accepting the diploma while shaking the dean's hand. Then (*and this is important*), write down several steps you can take to start making progress. In this example, it may be this:

1. Research and decide on which college/program
2. Plan when to take each class and how long it will take to complete the degree
3. Register and start taking classes
4. Schedule time Monday, Tuesday and Thursday evenings for study time

ACTION STEPS

1.

2.

3.

4.

5.

6.

7.

8.

9.

10.

When you have goals written down, you are much more likely to make progress toward them. Just moving forward boosts your faith in yourself and God, which lifts your mood and makes you more likely to achieve your goal. We read in Habakkuk, "And then GOD answered: 'Write this. Write what you see. Write it out in big block letters so that it can be read on the run. This vision-message is a witness pointing to what's coming. It aches for the coming—it can hardly wait! And it doesn't lie. If it seems slow in coming, wait. It's on its way. It will come right on time" (Habakkuk 2:2–3 The Message). The New King James says, "Write the vision and make it plain on tablets." What is a tablet? How about a journal? Business coaches and life coaches are huge proponents of writing goals down. I love the Message version telling us to write it out in big block letters! Make your goals plain and easy to see, and purposely look at them often. Then when you are aching to see results, you can ensure you are doing something to move forward, you'll be excited to wait, and your faith will be strengthened.

You know the saying that God helps those who help themselves? God gives us tools and techniques, and then He strengthens us to take advantage of them. Take authority over your circumstances and start to dream. *It's okay to dream big!* Stay close to God and allow Him to make your life what He wants it to be. He will give you the desires of your heart. "Delight yourself also in the LORD, and He shall give you the desires of your heart" (Psalm 37:4). He may adjust your desire to be more in line with His, but don't fret—He loves to give us good gifts! Start dreaming and get those goals in your journal.

Face Your Fears

Anxiety is rampant in our modern society. Many people struggle with unease and fear, which robs them of peace and joy. While people try desperately to suppress their fears, you won't overcome until you face them. Don't be afraid to really think about your deepest fears. This is where you gain the power to truly overcome. Anxiety is living in fear of something bad happening. Sometimes the fear is real, if you live with an abusive and unpredictable partner. But sometimes it is ridiculous, like being afraid your graduating senior is going to go away to college and not need you anymore. No matter what it is, the fear is like a clever bully, whispering into your ear. It never comes right into your field of view and screams at you. It is sneaky and makes you feel edgy and unsettled, and you aren't even sure why.

We must learn that the best way to deal with a bully is to confront them loudly and with confidence. The song "Fear is a Liar" by Zach Williams is powerful. The chorus reminds us that fear is a liar, stealing happiness and needing to be cast into the fire. If you struggle with anxiety, look up the lyrics for the verses and listen to this song on repeat. It is a list of lies the enemy tells us, which we can overcome by intentionally using our faith.

When you are praying or journaling, start writing down a list of your fears. Write down small things and big things. Here's an example:

> » I'll have a stroke and can't work, and then we'll run out of money.
>
> » I'll get cancer and die.
>
> » My son will die in a car crash because he is a new driver.

> » I will lose my job and become homeless.

> » My sister will get sick and die.

> » My house will burn up in a fire or be destroyed in a hurricane.

FEARS

Now you have a choice: Continue to live with fear and anxiety, or face your fears and think through how you would deal with those situations. It's up to you. One of the most powerful sermons I have ever heard was by Stephen Furtick of Elevation Church. His book *Chatterbox* is packed full of strategies to defeat negative self-talk. He tells the story of a family whose worst nightmare came true. Their three-year-old son died suddenly. Their world suddenly was forever different, and they were in shock. Furtick compared it to falling down a deep well.[49] One minute you are walking in the sunshine, then suddenly you are deep down a dark well. You have no idea why it happened or what you are going to do. You may even want to die.

But you can choose to realize that God is right there with you. Like the Hebrews in the fire or Daniel in the lions' den, God is with you in the worst of times. Whatever the circumstances, He's there with you. You have to choose to believe that there is going to be some way He will use it in your life. And know that God will be with you every moment as the healing and rebuilding slowly come.

Often just facing your fears and planning what you would do if they happened takes a lot of the fear away. Years ago, our son had several bad seizures that required him to be treated in the ICU. Because of that experience, I've had to face my worst-case-scenario fears. If my son has another severe seizure and passes away, it would be unspeakably awful, but I know we have a large group of family and friends that would be by our side helping us walk through it. I know that we would do something in his memory to help other special needs children. Thinking about the fear of losing my son paves the way for thinking about the action steps we could take to support other families experiencing similar circumstances and how we would cope and heal, and that gives me some peace.

Recently, I had to bring up a subject with my husband, Bill, that I knew wasn't going to be a comfortable discussion. I was afraid because of how previous similar discussions had gone. We've been married over twenty years and have learned what our hot button issues are after this long! I put off the discussion for a few days, blaming it on being tired, stressed, and other such things. I realized one morning that I was allowing my fear to control me. *(Head slap.)* I made myself think through the negative things I was afraid could happen, and then I allowed myself to plan how I would respond. I felt empowered by having faced my fears. I knew how I would respond if he didn't like my idea.

That night we finally talked, and my fears were unfounded. He totally understood my thoughts and supported my decision. I can't help but wonder how often I have been paralyzed by fear. Peter was writing to me, "Stay alert! Watch out for your great enemy, the devil. He prowls around like a roaring lion, looking for someone to devour. Stand firm against him, and be strong in your faith" (1 Peter 5:8-9 NLT). I need to remember Paul's words as well: "For God has not given us a spirit of fear, but of power and of love and of a strong mind" (2 Timothy 1:7).

We need to realize that fear is the enemy. John writes, "There is no fear in love; but perfect love casts out fear, because fear involves torment. But he who fears has not been made perfect in love" (1 John 4:18). God is peace and faith. When you fear, you are giving your enemy power over your thoughts. *Don't do it!* If the enemy tries to afflict you with sickness that is not of God, know that He will give you the tools to fight it and get the victory. If he wants you to stay healthy and live a vibrant life until you're ninety-eight, it's going to happen. We need to trust God. He will not allow you to go through more than that you can overcome. He gives us faith and the Word, which are both powerful weapons we can use against fear and circumstances. Don't fear the trials you face . . . face them boldly and grow through them.

One more note on facing fears—*stop speaking them!* There is a very powerful spiritual principle about the power that comes through the spoken word. When you speak positive things, it creates a channel for the Spirit to move through to make good things happen. But if you speak negative things, you immediately shut the channel down. If it is raining when you wake up Saturday morning, don't say, "*Rats.* It's raining. Guess we can't go to the beach." Instead, speak no doubt. Command the rain to stop, and then the sun just may come out! If God spoke the world into existence, and God's spirit lives in you, you have the creative power of God within you. Toby Mac's song "Speak Life" alludes to this. Give this song a listen!

Your words have the same power in them to create as God's words had during Creation. You can speak faith, speak hope, speak gratitude, and speak joy in all circumstances. It's not always easy, especially when you aren't particularly feeling those things, but that's actually part of the secret. When you speak faith, your faith will lift a bit. Speak it again, and you'll have more faith. Speak hope and expectation, and you'll feel it more. Speak joy, and you won't be as discouraged. It may take time and repetition, but fear will subside the more you speak faith. I promise!

I also encourage you to check your spirit throughout the day. I have had more than a few patients over the years that lived a life filled with anxiety. They are the ones who come in with a long list of symptoms for which they claim that nothing has worked. These visits are challenging, not only because I often struggle to offer a course of treatment that is acceptable, but honestly because these people often don't listen. They are much more comfortable living in a world of anxious thoughts than pushing them aside to focus on something or someone else.

When you are filled with anxiety, it becomes your focus. You cannot see outside yourself. It's amazing to me how often a spouse is drawn into the whirlwind of a patient's anxiety. The spouse is attentive and tries to help in any way possible, and the patient feeds off the attention and then becomes more self-centered. They both completely miss out on the great big world out there. Anxiety is just plain selfish! Paul reminds us, "Let each of you look out not only for his own interests, but also for the interests of others" (Philippians 2:4) and again in Romans, "For those who live according to the flesh set their minds on the things of the flesh, but those who live according to the Spirit, the things of the Spirit. For to be carnally minded is death, but to be spiritually minded is life and peace" (Romans 8:5–6).

When you are worried about yourself, are you thinking how to give to others? How to make someone else's life better? How to grow in your faith? I think not.

Closely related to fear is the uncertainty of doubt. The main reason people doubt is that they are afraid to fully believe. Think about how you feel when you hear a marketing pitch that sounds great, but you know it sounds too good to be true. You doubt what it is claiming. You are operating out of an appropriate sense of concern that if you trust it and purchase the item, you will be scammed and regret it. We have been so conditioned to distrust marketers, politicians and government officials, that we distrust even things that God is trying to do for us. God presents an opportunity, and our skeptical self comes out. We fear that God won't do it, and we will be disappointed or look stupid for believing.

I had an experience as a brand-new believer way back in college. I had been saved only a few months and was totally soaking in the Word and enjoying the new believer's high, but I was green in my faith and hadn't had it tested too much. I went to a summer camp meeting with friends, and a well-known, powerful preacher was preaching the evening services. He was well known for ministering to people at the altar and praying for their healing. Sure enough, one night he prayed for many people to be healed, and based on their immediate reactions, it seemed that most of them were receiving healing. Although I was too timid to go up to be prayed for, I prayed in my seat for healing from the asthma that had plagued me for years. I felt a powerful touch of the Spirit and felt like maybe, *just maybe,* I was healed, too! But after service, you guessed it, my lungs started to feel that familiar tightness. I felt like I had completely been made a fool. The enemy started telling me that I wasn't good enough to be healed, that I really didn't pray right, and that healing wasn't for me. I remember walking around the campground by myself and then just sitting down and crying.

It took me years to see that it wasn't my fault at all, but it was a lesson God was trying to teach me. The enemy absolutely loves to throw roadblocks in our way to make us doubt God's love and his power. I fell for it back then—*hook, line and sinker.* When we fight battles and seem to not get what we pray for, we often just give up. Instead, it should strengthen our faith. We are to continue to believe in God for healing, by standing on His promises in the Word. Honestly, God can use us even more powerfully if we press through without giving up. Don't doubt or fear. *Believe!* Note: it took me years to figure out exactly why I had asthma growing up. The journey to healing was long but taught me much as an integrative physician, and as I achieved healing, I was able to take what I learned and use it to help my patients heal in many ways. God can use even your failures.

Doubt is fearing that God can't do it. Doubt is fearing that God doesn't want to do it. Doubt is fearing that God doesn't want to do it for you. Doubt is simply fear.

Remember the story of the disciples in the storm? Jesus was asleep in the stern of the boat. The storm suddenly rose up, the boat was covered in waves, and the disciples fully believed they were about to die! They were experienced with boating, so this must have been a horrible storm. But Jesus kept sleeping. Think about that. The disciples must have been saying, *"Are you kidding me? Sleeping? He's not even helping us keep this boat afloat!"* Finally, they woke him up, saying, *"We are dying! Don't you care? Save us!"*

In these words, they showed how fearful they were and how much faith they were placing in their circumstances instead of in Him. Fear is choosing to believe what you see, not God—and is the opposite of the faith we should have, "Now faith is the substance of things hoped for, the evidence of things not seen" (Hebrews 11:1). Doubt is succumbing to fear. What did Jesus say to them? "Why are you so fearful? How is it that you have no faith?" (Mark 4:40). It's like he's saying, *"Really? Zero faith, guys? Haven't you learned anything I've taught you?"* What a rebuke.

When my son Daniel still had terrible seizures, I remember the first time I had to ride in the ambulance with him. This was his first seizure that wouldn't stop (status epilepticus). We had been in the ER for a while and despite all the meds they tried, they had to put him on the ventilator with sedation. Now that time, I was scared. We were riding in the ambulance from the first hospital to the children's hospital where he was going to be admitted. Several nurses were in back with my child on a ventilator, and I rode up front. It was very odd riding along in a quiet ambulance. No siren, no rushing, we just leisurely drove through traffic with my son in the back. In that moment, I knew with all my medical training that he could die. Not necessarily from the seizure, but complications of prolonged seizures can include kidney failure, pneumonia, and infection. It was a moment I'll never forget. I felt the presence of God so strongly riding in the front of that ambulance. Some of you have had this kind of experience. I just knew that God was there, I knew He was in control, and I knew that it would be okay if He took my son. I chose to let go of fear and let God be in control. I chose to face my fear of death, and I knew that if my son died, I would choose to rejoice in a life so full of blessings. My son has a special ability to create joy in others. Sure, he has his meltdowns that can be horrible. But he has such a sense of humor, too! He loves to be silly with his iPad or with videos he watches online, and he loves it when we are silly with him. When he smiles, you can't help but feel joy. I knew that if he died, we could be overwhelmed with thankfulness for the time we had with him and all the lives he touched.

Thankfully, he pulled through, and then he's had the same thing happen several times since then. We continue to trust God for his health and his future. You must celebrate the good, even when it is mixed in with bad stuff. We can choose thankfulness over fear and doubt.

Gratefulness

One of my favorite TED talks is by David Steindl-Rast, called "Want to be happy? Be grateful." He is a monk who talks about being present in the moment and being grateful for the many things we not only aren't grateful for, but we don't even notice. He reminds us that every day is a new gift. Have you even seen the videos of a child getting a hearing implant for the first time? They suddenly have a brand-new sense to enjoy, and their wonder and appreciation for sound is pure heavenly joy. We can experience that same joy of gratefulness every day. Steindl-Rast talks about viewing each day as "this unique day." He says: "If you learn to respond as if it were the first day win your life and the very last day, then you will have spent this day very well. Open your heart to all these blessings and let them flow through you, that everyone whom you will meet on the street will be blessed by you, just by your eyes, by your smile, by your touch, just by your presence. Let the gratefulness overflow into blessing all around you. Then it will really be a good day."[50]

When was the last time you gazed up at the clouds and really looked at them? When did you last admire a sunset filled with orange and pink? Do you really look at the flowers out in your yard, or do you not even notice them now? Are you grateful for the breeze when you are walking your dog? Are you grateful that you have air conditioning on a hot, humid summer day? What about the soft blanket you use when you are sitting on the couch on a chilly night? There are so many things we should be grateful for.

GRATITUDE LIST

I got upset this morning because the ice dispenser on our refrigerator malfunctioned. I was trying to get ice, and it was whirring and moving, but no ice came out. I gave up and then opened the freezer to look at it, and then all that ice came pouring out all over me and the floor. There was a jam in the dispenser. I was grumbling for a few minutes, cleaning up ice and water all over the kitchen floor. But if my biggest problem is picking up ice from an ice maker that makes my drink cold, I have it pretty good! I don't have cancer, my kids aren't on drugs, and my extended family are all happy and healthy. What's there to complain about, really?

Last month was another perfect example of choosing to be thankful. Daniel's seizures are benign now, but as I mentioned, in the past they were severe. Several times he had to be admitted to ICU and put on a ventilator with powerful sedatives just to get the seizures to stop. The last time he was admitted, my husband and I were sitting on the small couch in his hospital room. Daniel was on the ventilator with IVs and cords snaked all over his bed, as was usual then. We were laughing and giggling over something when the nurse came in. She looked at us and commented that we were very relaxed for the situation we were in. We explained that after the third or fourth time going through it, we didn't panic anymore. We trusted God was in control. She was so used to parents with high anxiety and fear. But she was thankful, because our lack of anxiety made her job so much easier.

Last month, Daniel was sitting at the kitchen table about to eat his eggs. He grabbed his head and wasn't acting right, and I realized he was going to have a seizure. I was able to get him up, walk him to the couch, and take his glasses off—just in time. He then had a typical seizure. Afterward, I was just so grateful for two things. First, he gave me enough warning that he was able to walk to the couch. When a teenager has a seizure at the kitchen table, all you can do is get them on the floor. Having the seizure on the couch was a huge blessing. Second, it was a normal seizure which stopped within five minutes. No ambulance needed.

Most people would be full of anxiety and frustration when this happens. Worried about complications, frustrated because they can't go to work, and always worried about when he'll have another one and if it would be a big one with deadly complications. Instead, I chose to be thankful. Thankful that my child would sleep it off and be fine in a few hours. Thankful that I have staff in my office who can cover for me at the office. Thankful that my child is such a great gift to me and those who know him.

You can always find something to be grateful for. I believe God allows trials to come not only to shape our character and increase our trust in Him, but to challenge us to look for the good. For example, if you grow up rich, it's harder to appreciate what you have. When I was growing up, we only went clothes shopping once a year in August for school. We could only get a few shirts and a few pairs of pants, but we cherished them! New clothes were a special treat, and we appreciated them. When is the last time you looked at your closet and were thankful? I remember in college when we were all poor. We found an old couch on the curb, and we were so grateful to have it! We knew that the shabby furniture we had was functional and within our budget, so we appreciated it. We didn't focus on the fact that it was used, an ugly color, or not stylish. We focused on the good, not the bad.

When that poison ivy finally goes away, you are thankful for healthy skin.

When the power goes out for an evening, you are thankful when you have light and HVAC again.

When you come home from camping, you are thankful for a hot shower and clean clothes.

When ______,

I am thankful for ______.

When ______,

I am thankful for ______.

When ______,

I am thankful for ______.

Don't fall for the lie that gratefulness is a result of happiness or having what you want. It's the opposite; being happy is a result of being grateful. Paul reminds us, "In everything give thanks; for this is the will of God in Christ Jesus for you" (1 Thessalonians 5:18). This is not for all things, but in all things. If you have health, breath, family, and friends, you are abundantly blessed. Philippians 4:8 tells us to think and meditate on things that are true, noble, just, pure, lovely, and of good report. That sounds like gratefulness to me.

One more thing you can do to feel better is to give. We all know what joy it brings to give gifts to others! At least, I hope you do! If you are feeling down, find something you can give, whether it is money, items to charity, a meal for a neighbor, or your time. To further your joy, find a way to give something of value to someone anonymously. It's so much fun to do! One year, we adopted a family at church and bought gifts for the whole family. It was better than getting presents! Luke says, "Give, and it will be given to you: good measure, pressed down, shaken together, and running over will be put into your bosom" (Luke 6:38). You will get much more back than you give.

Exercise

While exercise is obviously physical, it has amazing psychological benefits. We all know exercise helps the body deal with stress. Those of you who work out know what I'm saying is true. When you finish a good workout, your brain feels better. Sure, your muscles also get stronger, but there is truly a brain boosting effect. Several things happen with exercise, one of which is that it boosts dopamine. Dopamine is the neurotransmitter that causes a feeling of reward and pleasure. When you finish cleaning out the garage, you're tired and sweaty, but it looks amazing, and your brain is filled with dopamine. You feel a sense of pride, accomplishment, and completion which gives you pleasure. This makes you much more stress resilient. Testosterone also goes up after working out. That, too, boosts your moods and your motivation to do things.

Those that exercise regularly are more resilient to stress and the physical changes it causes. Mentally, things don't bother you as much. Your moods are better. You aren't as tired and can handle complex situations with a better attitude. Even if the stressful situation doesn't change, your response to it is dramatically better.

If you are busy from dawn to dusk, you may not have time to exercise. You're too tired or too busy in the evening to go to the gym. Saturdays are now filled with more activities outside of the house and less with raking leaves or washing the windows like we did when I was growing up. We drive everywhere and sit all day long, especially for those that work from home. When is the last time you parked in the furthest parking spot at the store and walked all the way across the lot for exercise? How often do you take the stairs, other than to your second-floor bedroom? In general, as a society, we have become sedentary.

Different types of exercise have different effects. Aerobic exercise (cardio) will help you burn off steam. It can be exhausting, but in a good way. Weightlifting gives you an energizing sense of strength. Playing a sport is just generally fun and doesn't feel like work, so think about how you can incorporate more sporting activities. Consider taking up something new. My sister introduced me to pickleball recently. I now understand its explosive growth! Several of my patients in their sixties play pickleball, because it gives you a nice blend of mild cardio, range of motion, core strength, and social fun. It's a great stress reducer!

Team sports bring a sense of community to exercise, and the results can be tremendous in terms of dealing with stress. Even going to the gym with a workout partner or playing golf with others is much more fun than doing it alone. I also know a couple that has been ballroom dancing for years. They do it regularly and are very good, and I would argue it has helped their marriage be so successful. Exercise is good for your health, your stress, and your relationships!

Yoga is a special exercise associated with stress relief. It's been studied a lot, and numerous studies have shown that those who do yoga regularly have better cortisol levels.[51] Yoga also has been shown to reduce depression and symptoms of PTSD and improve sleep.[52]

Lastly, just walking is not *just* anything. While a leisurely stroll is not enough to help you lose weight, it is great at reducing stress. Walking stretches out your body and gets your blood flowing. It improves circulation to the brain, which helps it reboot. Getting outside to breathe fresh air (if you don't live in the heart of the city) is also so good for you. Sunshine helps too, especially the infrared rays of the late afternoon. Another good time to walk is in the morning. If you get sunlight on your face first thing in the morning, the light stimulates your brain to wake up. Even Hippocrates said, "Walking is a natural exercise, much more so than the other exercises," and he also says that "a walk after dinner dries the belly and body; it prevents the stomach becoming fat."[53] This makes me laugh! Get out there and get moving, whether it's walking or a sport. It's important!

Counseling

Counseling can also be a very powerful strategy in dealing with stress. We all need to realize that we are not very objective about ourselves. We tend to only see our point of view, especially when emotions are involved. If someone hurts you, you only feel your pain and feel wronged. It's very hard to consider the reasons why the person hurt you. Maybe they are going through something stressful themselves, and they are taking it out on others unwittingly. Sometimes people are just ignorant and have no idea how their words or behavior are perceived by others.

Counselors or therapists have a great ability to help you see your situation more clearly. Having a neutral person work through your thoughts with you helps you know which of your observations are true and which are not true. They also help you identify your feelings and work through them. Quite often, our feelings are not based on accurate facts and need to be redirected or reframed. Sometimes they are dangerous, because they lead us to do and say things that make things a lot worse. Have you ever had a stupid argument with a family member over something and then realized later that it wasn't even worth arguing about? We lack perspective sometimes and can be overcome by emotion. We need help identifying what is or isn't true and sorting through our emotions. Only then can we make good choices about what to do next.

Early in our marriage, my husband and I went through some rough times. We were just terrible at communicating our feelings. Well, in all fairness, *I* was terrible at communicating my feelings. He was good at letting me know how he felt; he just did it in an angry way that made me withdraw. We had a lot of arguments. I was seeing a counselor at the time, and she helped me realize that his anger was in response to my withdrawing. He had a fear of rejection, and I was adding to it by not talking—which resulted in him responding with anger. I had to learn to communicate a lot better and reassure him I wasn't going anywhere. He had to learn to not listen to that voice in his head creating fear, and we both learned how to be better communicators. Counseling helped each of us realize this important fact: my spouse is not like me, and he or she thinks differently. What a revelation, right? It's amazing what you can learn about yourself when someone gives you an objective assessment.

If you have not yet read *The Five Love Languages* by Gary Chapman, you need to. This book has changed the lives of millions since it was first published. If you have any problems communicating and connecting with your spouse or children, you need to read it. The main concept is that we all have certain ways that communicate love powerfully to us.[54] If someone loves us in their language instead of in ours, it doesn't make us feel as loved. My husband's primary love language is quality time. Mine is acts of service. If I cook a fancy supper and then clean up the kitchen until it is spotless, I feel like I'm really loving him by blessing him. But he feels unloved because I spent so much time cooking and cleaning up when I could have been spending time with him. He would feel much more loved if I cooked something quick and simple, had time to sit with him while dinner was cooking, and then let the dishes pile up while we sat after dinner and talked over a cup of tea. That time together speaks more love to him than anything I do for him. You need to learn to love your family members in the way they feel most loved, even if it's not your love language.

Learning more about yourself and your family goes a long way toward dealing with stressful situations. If you are having problems with a teenager, counseling is a must. Teens just don't naturally open up totally with their parents. That's okay! If you haven't started counseling because you are afraid of not finding someone you feel comfortable with or think it's going to require weekly sessions, I encourage you to just schedule the first appointment. Like any other medical or professional service, if you don't feel like it's a good fit after a session or two, you don't need to go back. Find someone else. Most of the time, you will meet with the counselor for a month or two regularly, but then you can space out your sessions. Don't assume you're going to be stuck in counseling for a long time. If you need it long-term, definitely continue. But a lot of people just need help for a while until they grow through a tough situation and overcome it.

There is nothing wrong with seeing a counselor indefinitely as a preventive measure. I knew a wonderful Christian couple in their early sixties. They had been in ministry for decades and were some of the kindest, most giving people I've ever known. She told me over lunch how they see a counselor once a month as a marriage tune-up. They never argued and had never had severe issues, but that once-a-month session helped them address little things before they could become a threat. I was so surprised and so impressed!

If you ever feel like you are being coerced or manipulated emotionally, please seek professional help. It is never okay for others to make you feel like your feelings, thoughts or opinions don't matter and aren't valid. Others can disagree with you, but if you feel afraid to express yourself due to fear of reprisal, something isn't right. Emotional boundaries are essential to a healthy sense of self and to healthy relationships. Abuse often starts very subtly but can escalate quickly. Counseling can help you see your situation more clearly and address issues in the best way possible, even if it means making hard decisions.

When you learn good emotional boundaries, you own your emotions and thoughts, and you are less likely to be affected by others' negative emotions. Codependency can result when you are always worried about making other people happy and you feel responsible for their well-being. When they are angry or depressed, you take those emotions on as well. This may be true for you and your spouse, but it also happens with parents and their children. This is a miserable way to live.

If you struggle with pleasing others at the expense of yourself, sacrificing your own wants and needs, or even blaming others for your problems, it's important to work through this with a counselor. If you're having trouble parenting a strong-willed child, talking to a counselor who is objective can give you a new perspective and equip you with good ideas about how to unemotionally impose consequences and discipline. Don't be afraid to seek out a wise counselor to walk with you through tough issues. Counselors are there for *you*.

If, for some reason, you choose not to see a therapist, an alternative is to seek out a mentor or accountability partner. When I was newly married, I was close to a few older women in church who were a good sounding board for me. Older women (or older men, if you're a male) have wisdom and experience and can give godly advice. Having a friend as an accountability partner is also valuable. If you tell your friend that you are going to go to the gym three days in a week or that you want to stop eating cookies, they can check in and ask you how you're doing with your goals. You are more likely to follow through if you know someone is going to ask you about it. Think about being in school. How many optional assignments did you do? Probably not a lot. The work you did was because the teacher was going to ask you for it. Weight loss programs that work usually have accountability in them. A weight loss coach or fellow dieters asking you how you did that week is a powerful motivator!

Whether your stress is big or little, if you feel like you aren't handling it well or it is affecting your life significantly, I encourage you to talk to someone regularly. There is a powerful effect in just venting and communicating your feelings. Like journaling, getting things out by talking to someone else often helps us work through things, and we feel more capable to handle the situation. I read a book years ago called *The Red Tent* by Anita Diamant. It is a fictional book about Dinah, a daughter of Jacob. She grows up around her mother, Leah, as well as Rachel, Zilpah, and Bilhah. The red tent was where women went during their period when they were considered unclean. It was a place where women connected and learned from each other. Older women counseling younger women. Women teaching and connecting with other women. Men are also called to connect with each other. My husband and the other men in our church's men's group go out for breakfast every Saturday morning. They connect as men, sharing their struggles and victories, and encouraging and teaching each other. Connection and community are what makes us strong!

Hobbies

Everyone has things they do to help relieve stress, such as playing tennis, making gourmet food, listening to music, or in my case, knitting. I tried several times as a teenager to learn how to knit, since all my female relatives were knitters. I couldn't get it, and for years I wanted to learn. A few years ago, I was determined to learn. It took a few weeks, but I did it! Anyone who knits or crochets will tell you that it is very calming and enjoyable.

I've mentioned the recent craze for pickleball. I don't know anyone who has tried it and hasn't liked it. If there are courts or leagues in your area, consider giving it a try! We also live near a lake, and people around here love to go boating or fishing. You don't need a lot of money for a used fishing pole. Find a good spot and get up early. But there are an infinite number of things you can do for fun. Here are some, but this is just scratching the surface:

- » Play golf. (Even mini golf is easy to fit in and a great social connection!)

- » Volunteer at a community organization. (A great one for stress relief is a local animal shelter!)

- » Build or refinish furniture. (There are lots of good cheap finds at yard sales that, with some TLC, can be totally renovated and then used, given away, or sold.)

- » Play cards. (This seems to be a dying art, and I'm not sure a smoky poker game with beer is the healthiest thing, but playing cards with friends can be a lot of fun.)

- » Make art: painting, whittling/carving, making jewelry, making decorative painted signs (home decor)

- » Learn to arrange flowers. Fishing and hunting

- » Make soap or scented bath salts.

- » Put together a jigsaw puzzle.

- » Collect coins.

- » Go canoeing or kayaking.

- » Learn to cook. (Start a neighborhood *gourmet* group, where each month you cook an ethnically themed meal.)

- » Get outside and go camping.

- » Learn to play the guitar or piano.

- » Learn to bake. (Learn how to make a complicated dessert and you'll have a lot of fun giving them for gifts.)

If you have a current hobby, and you're not spending time enjoying it, schedule time for it. As I've mentioned a few times, you generally don't just end up in the middle of the day with unexpected free time. You will probably have to schedule time, but it will be worth it! Whether it's a Saturday afternoon or a Tuesday evening, just schedule a small amount of time. You're never too busy to do a little something fun.

If you don't have any current hobbies, consider things you've done in the past. Did you used to play a sport years ago? Maybe you can find a recreational adult league. What about a rusty musical skill that you could brush up on? Anything that you used to enjoy is worth consideration. But feel free to explore and find something new to try. Don't be afraid to be a beginner! Learning a new skill is not only a stressbuster, but good for your brain, especially if you are over forty. We tend to get comfortable in the things we do and are good at, but learning new skills helps our cognitive function and stress adaptation response. This can improve your performance in your job. Hobbies can help improve your memory, concentration and focus and improves your fine motor skills and hand-eye coordination.

Hobbies also just make you a more interesting person to be around and often boost your overall confidence and self-esteem. You feel better about yourself, you are connecting with others, and therefore, stress doesn't affect you as much. So have fun and play!

HOBBIES OR SKILLS TO LEARN

Self-care

As we've discussed earlier in this book, self-care is essential. The Bible acknowledges that it is completely natural for us to care for ourselves: "You shall love your neighbor as yourself" (Mark 12:31). This means that we naturally seek comfort and relief from stress. Unfortunately, if it's not balanced by work and responsibility, it can lead to failure. There are healthy and not-so-healthy ways to relax and de-stress. Chocolate, wine, and binge-watching shows may be okay occasionally, but it will be hard to succeed in life if you indulge in them every day.

Many of us find it very hard to stop and care for ourselves. Every day that I see patients, I find myself encouraging them to slow down and focus some time on themselves. Men often work from the time they get up until they come home, and often continue to work on something at night without relaxing with their family. Women are so good at taking care of everyone else that we also often find it hard to sit and relax.

Again, when was the last time you simply sat down on the couch and did nothing but relax? What about sitting outside to watch the sun go down? If it's been a while, you're typical. We generally either go to work, or we have a list of things we need to work on if we aren't working. I think a lot of us are pretty good at relaxing on the weekends, but even then, sometimes we are adding to our stress because we are still doing things with family and going places.

When was the last time you were truly relaxed and rejuvenated? For me, it was at a conference I was recently attending. I am not a spa person and have never before missed conference sessions for the spa, but I did it this time. I spent a heavenly hour in the spa getting a massage and it was just wonderful. It felt like a totally unnecessary, expensive thing to do (and wrong in the sense that I missed an hour of the conference). But afterward, I realized how important it is to purposefully make time in my busy schedule for relaxation.

Do you have time at work to go outside for a fifteen-minute walk at lunch? Can you take a walk in your neighborhood when you first get home from work? Can you take a short bath in the evening to reboot your brain for the evening? Think about ways to pamper yourself a bit. Certainly, all things should be in moderation, so don't go busting your budget on splurges that make you feel good but leave no room for other family needs. A little self-nurturing will go a long way.

Self-nurturing helps you realize that you are worth it. Instead of seeing all your flaws and failures, you will start to see yourself more positively. You will see yourself how God sees you—filled with unique attributes and strengths, completely worthy of being loved, and blessed beyond measure. God loves you, so you need to love you, too!

SELF-CARE IDEAS

Assess your Situation

One of the most important things you need to do when you are stressed out is to do a thorough assessment of what things you have any control over and what you cannot control. For example, your attitude is totally up to you. But other people's behavior is not at all something you can control.

CONTROLLABLE	NOT CONTROLLABLE
» Your thoughts	» Other people's thoughts
» Your emotions, to a degree	» Other people's emotions
» Your speech	» Other people's speech
» Your actions	» Other people's actions
» Your family	» Weather
» Your job	» Your boss's actions
» Volunteering/ministry	» Church leadership
» Where you live	» Other people's personality
» How often you talk to or visit family	» Your family's behavior
» Your church	» Your neighbors

When my one of my sons was a teenager, he was a handful! He went through a phase in his mid-teens when he didn't want to shower and was a total slob. His room, *oh boy!* It was a disaster all the time, and it did not smell good. He would leave clothes all over the floor, and he would stash candy wrappers and dirty dishes under the bed—*it was gross.* Yelling at him wasn't doing any good. We were not able to make him care that he stunk and his room was a pig sty. It just wasn't important to him. We had to realize the following:

> » Yelling wasn't doing anything.
>
> » We had no control over how he felt about it or how he acted in response.

» We had no way to make him see it our way or convince him. That just wasn't happening.

» We did have control over what he was required to do as a bare minimum.

» We were able to set firm rules and boundaries. (For example, if we found dirty dishes in his room, he had dish duty every day for a week. He also had to shower at least once a day—non-negotiable.)

» We chose to not get upset *at all*. We simply stated the rules and the consequences *without emotion*.

It worked! It took a while for him to mature and learn how to keep clutter at bay, but it eventually happened. It just wasn't a battle worth yelling about and stressing ourselves over. Bypass the fights and the stress, and keep your cool. It's much easier that way.

I challenge you to ask yourself, how much of this stress I'm feeling is caused by me? If I didn't cause it, am I increasing it because of my reaction? Even if I'm not adding to it, am I prolonging it because of how I'm acting? If your actions have any part in the stress, you and *you alone* are responsible for your part in it.

On the other hand, if the situation is not something you are contributing to, you need to accept that and let it go. Consider that someone you love has cancer—that's clearly no one's fault. Your job is to stand in faith and find some good in it.

Remember the Serenity prayer?

> *God, give me grace to accept with serenity*
> *the things that cannot be changed,*
> *Courage to change the things*
> *which should be changed,*
> *and the Wisdom to distinguish*
> *the one from the other.*

> *Living one day at a time,*
> *Enjoying one moment at a time,*

Accepting hardship as a pathway to peace,
Taking, as Jesus did,
This sinful world as it is,
Not as I would have it,
Trusting that You will make all things right,
If I surrender to Your will,
So that I may be reasonably happy in this life,
And supremely happy with You forever in the next. Amen.

—Reinhold Niebuhr[55]

I challenge you to simply examine all your stress for a week in light of this poem. What can you change? What can't you change? The most common mistake we make is underestimating how powerful we are to change our thoughts and actions. And for the things we cannot control, like other people, choose to love them with the love of God and not let them pull you down. Vow to not ruminate about things you cannot control. Let God use those things that are out of your control to mold you, smooth your rough edges, and make you better.

CONTROLLABLE   **NOT CONTROLLABLE**

Choose How to Respond

You have full control over how you respond to situations. This is perhaps one of the biggest take home messages in this book. You cannot control what happens to you or what anyone else does. But you totally control your response! So many people respond poorly to stress. We whine, we blame others for our own unhappiness, and we feel sorry for ourselves, which makes us pretty unattractive. No one wants to be around a whiner who wallows in victimhood. We can rise above the stress simply by choosing to respond in a positive way using our faith.

Quit saying "I just had to" or "I couldn't help myself." Stop making excuses. Own up to any fault of yours that led to the stressful situation or the conflict. If you have made bad choices (like eating pizza and ice cream every Friday night or falling into a habit of avoiding prayer), don't be surprised when you aren't spiritually or physically healthy.

God will give you strength and direction. Choose to have a teachable spirit and a positive attitude, even if you are suffering. God's Spirit moves in such powerful ways when someone doesn't let suffering suppress their spirit. I've watched patients go through chemo with such joy and positivity that it put me to shame. I've seen patients in the hospital joking with nurses and ministering to the stressed-out staff, sharing Scriptures, or just an encouraging word. I've seen family members at a funeral do all they can to help someone else, even during their own grief. This is God's Spirit at work. When we allow Him to use us as a vessel of the Spirit, God accomplishes something.

Think about when a hurricane comes through an area and causes a lot of property damage. People come together to help neighbors out. After September 11, 2001, our country was united in a way that hadn't really happened since World War II. In times of stress, you stop bickering about dumb things and focus on the big picture. This is where God works. My friend, Linda, fought cancer for years. She was our babysitter for several years when my kids were young. She came to our house several days a week, proudly wearing her turban and dealing with more doctor and hospital visits than I could imagine. I really can't ever remember her being depressed, anxious, or irritable! She refused to be an emotional burden on other people. She insisted on continuing to minister and help other people. She was always the one volunteering at the church, even in between chemo appointments. She was my hero.

When you are emotionally and spiritually mature, you can separate your emotions from facts, and you make intentional choices on how you respond to hard situations. A good example of this are first responders and emergency department staff. Police, firefighters, doctors, and nurses all learn how to assess a critical situation and make quick, rational decisions on how to respond. Emotions are separated and are not part of the equation. One thing I learned in residency has stuck with me ever since. I was on a rotation with a pediatric neurologist, Warren Wasiewski, MD. He often saw children with epilepsy, so he dealt with seizures a lot. He taught all of us young residents that when a child is having a seizure, "Don't just do something; stand there." Say what? That's right, don't initially react. Our natural tendency is to let emotion or panic drive us to take action in haste. But the most important thing when someone is experiencing a seizure is to simply allow it to occur in a safe position. Sometimes that's also true with a stressful event. You just need to let it play out. If you get a flat tire on the way to work, don't allow emotional thoughts of anger or anxiety affect you. Decide whether you are going to put on the spare tire or call roadside assistance. Realize you're going to be late and accept it. Getting mad or full of anxiety will only ruin your day and affect the people you will be interacting with. Do your best and move on, and "having done all [you can], to stand [firm in faith]" (Ephesians 6:13, brackets added).

Remember this key concept for the rest of your life: You can't always control what happens around you or to you, but you have full control over your reaction to it.

CHAPTER 7

Spiritual Strategies for Healing

This is the beginning of the rest of the book. For science lovers, you've probably learned a lot about the biology of stress, and hopefully, you feel empowered to make needed changes. But for the believer, everything we have talked about so far actually pales in comparison to what we need to talk about next: *letting God heal us.*

When we are stressed, we are *diseased* in the sense that we are "dis" (not) at "ease." Our peace is disrupted. As Christians, we know that disease is the result of sin and the fall of man. Once Adam and Eve chose to eat of the forbidden fruit, disease entered the world. Generations of men lived under the curse of sin and disease for thousands of years until Jesus came to deliver us from that curse.

Man is born into sin and under the curse. This is why we need to be saved! If you are a new Christian, enjoy the adventure of learning from other Christians all about the amazing grace of God. What once was dead is now brought to life. Shame is eliminated, and we are filled with the power of God's love. We are no longer slaves to sin, but we walk in newness of life—"Knowing this, that our old man was crucified with Him, that the body of sin might be done away with, that we should no longer be slaves of sin" (Romans 6:6).

Many Christians stop there, however. They know that they are saved from sin and they live in God's grace. But they don't quite know or believe that they can be healed from disease, too. We are redeemed from the curse and have inherited the blessing of Abraham, which means full redemption from all aspects of the curse, *including disease*. We don't just have to accept sickness! God has given us a powerful weapon to use when sickness attacks us. But far too many of us just accept it and suffer through it, instead of getting victory.

Covenant of Abraham

The curse of sin brought about by Adam and Eve had far reaching consequences. Death and disease immediately came upon the earth, and they were driven out of the Garden of Eden. Strife, violence, fear, and pain were now a part of life.

When Abram was seventy-five years old, God told him to leave Haran with his family and go to Canaan. God promised him, "I will make you a great nation; I will bless you and make your name great; and you shall be a blessing" (Genesis 12:2). A few chapters later, God established His covenant with him.

> "When Abram was ninety-nine years old, the LORD appeared to Abram and said to him, 'I am Almighty God; walk before Me and be blameless. And I will make My covenant between Me and you, and will multiply you exceedingly.' Then Abram fell on his face, and God talked with him, saying: 'As for Me, behold, My covenant is with you, and you shall be a father of many nations. No longer shall your name be called Abram, but your name shall be Abraham; for I have made you a father of many nations. I will make you exceedingly fruitful; and I will make nations of you, and kings shall come from you. And I will establish My covenant between Me and you and your descendants after you in their generations, for an everlasting covenant, to be God to you and your descendants after you.'" —Genesis 17:1–7

The idea of a covenant isn't as meaningful to us as it was in Abraham's day. In modern times, we have contracts, lawyers, and courts because people violate contracts all the time, resulting in disputes. Back then, though, a covenant was simply a binding agreement that you did not break, *period.* When God covenanted with Abram, changing his name, it was a sure promise that He would do what He said!

Notice also how clear it is that this covenant would go on forever. The word translated "everlasting" means *forever, until eternity, perpetual.* It didn't die with Abraham.

Consider Moses and his final instructions to the Israelites when they were in Moab, after forty years in the wilderness, about to cross over into the promised land. The book of Deuteronomy is all about his instructions to the people. He knew that they were the chosen people of God and were about to inherit the land of milk and honey, but he also knew that they had issues with pride and rebellion. The entire book is Moses' advice to the people. He was warning them not to disobey God and encouraging them to receive the full blessing of their inheritance!

Deuteronomy 6:1–2 sums it up: "Now this is the commandment, and these are the statutes and judgments which the LORD your God has commanded to teach you, that you may observe them in the land which you are crossing over to possess, that you may fear the LORD your God, to keep all His statutes and His commandments which I command you, you and your son and your grandson, all the days of your life, and that your days may be prolonged."

I encourage you to read chapters 6–9 for yourself. Read them with the realization that not only are you adopted into the vine and part of God's holy people, but you are filled with the Spirit of God and wear the name of Jesus Christ. You belong in this chapter and have every right to all the blessings God showers on His people!

> "For you are a holy people to the LORD your God; the LORD your God has chosen you to be a people for Himself, a special treasure above all the peoples on the face of the earth . . . Therefore know that the LORD your God, He is God, the faithful God who keeps covenant and mercy for a thousand generations with those who love Him and keep His commandments." —Deuteronomy 7:6, 9

Consider just some of the blessings that God promises to his people:

- » His mercy
- » His love
- » His blessings
- » We will be multiplied
- » Our children will be blessed
- » Our land will be fruitful (businesses, homes)
- » No sickness
- » Power to get wealth
- » Plenty of food
- » Safe travel
- » Defeated enemies
- » Storehouses filled
- » Activities blessed
- » Esteem in the eyes of the world
- » Plenty of goods
- » We will lend and not borrow

You will find all of these in Deuteronomy 7, 8, and 28. Believe it or not, the blessing that started with Abraham and was preached to the Israelites included material wealth and physical health. You might be a little uncomfortable with that. Perhaps you have been taught that God allows His children to suffer poverty and sickness to bring us closer to Him or to strengthen us. While we can certainly grow closer to Him in times of suffering, do not believe the lie that it is God's will for us to suffer! We only need to look at the second half of Deuteronomy 28 to see why.

This is titled "Curses on Disobedience" in my Bible. Read verses 15 through 68. It's terrifying! The curses listed here cover everything from famine to sickness to slavery and more unspeakable things. My guess is that Moses knew some of the people were stubborn and needed to be told in explicit detail every bad thing that would happen if they forsook God. "Because you did not serve the LORD your God with joy and gladness of heart, for the abundance of everything, therefore you shall serve your enemies, whom the LORD will send against you, in hunger, in thirst, in nakedness, and in need of everything; and He will put a yoke of iron on your neck until He has destroyed you" (Deuteronomy 28:47–48).

Not only that, but sickness is clearly part of this curse: "Then the LORD will bring upon you and your descendants extraordinary plagues—great and prolonged plagues—and serious and prolonged sicknesses. Moreover He will bring back on you all the diseases of Egypt, of which you were afraid, and they shall cling to you. Also, every sickness and every plague, which is not written in the book of this law, will the LORD bring upon you until you are destroyed" (Deuteronomy 28:59–61).

Redemption From the Curse

That's the bad news. But what about the good news? We are redeemed from the curse! Galatians is a powerful book, and the secret to living in the blessings of God is found in chapters 3 and 4. We first read, "And the Scripture, foreseeing that God would justify the Gentiles by faith, preached the gospel to Abraham beforehand, saying 'In you all the nations shall be blessed'. So then those who are of faith are blessed with believing Abraham" (Galatians 3:8–9).

When we trust in God to save us and receive His grace, He cleanses us from sin and fills us with His Spirit in new life. This is because we place our faith in Him, not in ourselves or the world. Letting go fills us with His power and with true life. This is the beauty of salvation.

Salvation isn't just to receive forgiveness of sins and to call ourselves a Christian. It is to give us our inheritance! Salvation is the open door to God's riches. Sadly, many never really explore and receive all that God has for them. It's like being given the key to your rich father's safety deposit box at the bank after he passes away. You have the key to all his wealth, which you have just inherited, but if you don't go to the bank to access it, you will miss out on what you now own!

Jesus took on sin for us, carrying that curse to the cross and defeating it once and for all when he rose from the dead. "Christ has redeemed us from the curse of the law, having become a curse for us . . . that the blessing of Abraham might come upon the Gentiles in Christ Jesus, that we might receive the promise of the Spirit through faith" (Galatians 3:13–14).

We have inherited the blessing of Abraham! Every bit of the curse died with Christ on the cross and was destroyed when He rose again. All the blessings that Moses promised to the Israelites are now available to us. We are his chosen people! We are his children whom He loves intensely and wants to bless abundantly. We are actually "joint heirs with Christ" (Romans 8:17) because "as many of you as were baptized into Christ have put on Christ" (Galatians 3:27).

When we die to sin and are reborn into Christ, we are joined to Him in the Spirit. We become as much of an heir to the riches of God as Jesus! That is an amazing fact. We inherit everything that God has because we are now a part of His covenant with Abraham. "Therefore you are no longer a slave but a son, and if a son, then an heir of God through Christ" (Galatians 4:7)

Sickness is a result of sin and is from the enemy. God's will is healing and wellness. If you still don't believe me, take a few days and ask God to really speak to you about it. Read all these scriptures for yourself and pray about it. If you want to read more, I recommend *God's Will is Healing* by Gloria Copeland. You need to understand that we have every right to rebuke sickness and resist disease. I'm not saying sickness won't ever happen or it will be easy to defeat. We live in a fallen world that is teeming with toxins and stress that can cause disease easily. But just because the fight is difficult doesn't mean that we can give up and just accept it. Stand strong and use the Word to receive healing.

Once you understand that we don't have to accept sickness, you're ready to move forward to achieve healing. Remind yourself every day that "if you are Christ's, then you are Abraham's seed, and heirs according to the promise" (Galatians 3:29). Say it out loud to yourself: "Because I am Christ's, I am Abraham's seed, so I am an heir according to the promise of God!" With that expectation and that faith, you're ready to move on to strategies that will help you heal.

Repentance and Forgiveness

Before you can really receive God's restoration, the soil of your heart must be tilled and ready for it. This starts with repentance and forgiveness—both for yourself and for others. Repentance is not always easy, but it is necessary and powerful.

When you are starting a spiritual quest, seek the Lord first. Self-examine for any sin or disobedience in your heart. In Psalms, the Lord says, "I will guide you along the best pathway for your life. I will advise you and watch over you" (Psalm 32:8 NLT). I had a conversation once with a very close friend. I was discouraged at what seemed to be a lot of awful things happening in my life, and nothing was really working very well. She advised me to make sure there wasn't any sin I needed to repent, but also to make sure there wasn't something that God was waiting on me to do. I took it to heart and prayed about it. I didn't feel any conviction about sin, but I did realize what the problem was: *I was not working on this book!* This book has been several years in the making. I have some good reasons, and also some dumb excuses, for it taking a long time. Repent of anything that the Holy Spirit has been moving you to do that you haven't done.

If there is something you have failed to do, there is no condemnation in Christ. Acknowledge it in prayer and set your mind on your next steps to do it. Sometimes we miss out on the fullness of God's peace and joy simply because He's waiting on us to move. Repent of your inaction and move forward. But if it's more than that, and there is an element of sin, admit it and ask God to forgive you. He will! Receive his forgiveness and move forward in peace and power. Psalm 32 tells us, "Oh, what joy for those whose disobedience is forgiven, whose sin is put out of sight! Yes, what joy for those whose record the Lord has cleared of guilt, whose lives are live in complete honesty!" (Psalm 32:1–2 NLT).

Sometimes it's more than just inaction or even a particular area of sin. Unforgiveness is even worse because it creeps up on us so often below our awareness. Little offenses can add up over time and create deep emotional pain. Unforgiveness needs to be identified and taken care of early on. If not, it turns into deep bitterness, which is a malignancy on our spirit that seeks to destroy us. When we indulge it, we are sinning.

If you have bitterness in your heart, you need to be broken. It sounds harsh, but it is true. There is no way to live a victorious life while harboring pain and anger towards someone else. Bitterness is usually a result of having been wronged. One of the harsh realities of life is that it simply isn't fair. When many of us grew up, we learned this from our parents, our friends, and our life circumstances. We learned a degree of self-resilience because we had to accept that unfair things happen. We stood back up, got stronger, and moved forward.

Modern culture is different now. We live in a world of victims and offense. You can so easily offend some people by addressing them incorrectly, wearing a T-shirt with a controversial slogan, or even just looking at them wrong. There are many insecure, easily-offended people that live on the edge of anger and are quick to blame others for their misery. This is not God's will. Anyone who claims to be a believer and has a lifestyle of easy offense and anger is not right with God. God gave His life for our sins, and He forgives us. In return, He expects us to forgive others. If you are easily offended, I recommend reading the book *Unoffendable* by Brant Hansen. You'll see how ungodly it is to be offended. You'll repent and be forever changed!

But what about when you've been deeply hurt? When it's more than simply being offended, but you've been clearly wronged? It feels like you have every right to be angry and defensive. In the flesh, it feels good to be mad. You feel justified, because clearly, you were innocent, and they are guilty.

This is when it's so hard to let go. But you need to if you want to be free. I can assure you that emotional pain is completely normal and natural in these circumstances. Jesus hurt deeply when his disciples left him in the Garden of Gethsemane. I imagine him wanting to say, *"Really? You couldn't stay awake with me for one lousy hour when I'm about to give my life for you?"* He bore the sins of every person for all time when he was hanging on the cross. Believe me, he understands pain better than you or I ever will.

But we need to process the pain by forgiving and letting it go. On the cross, Jesus gave us the best example of how to do this, saying: "Father, forgive them, for they do not know what they do" (Luke 23:34). It's not always easy to have this attitude when someone hurts us, especially when they are our family and we can't easily separate from them, like we could a friend. But that's where the Holy Spirit comes in to help us.

God allows us to go through stress to mold us and change us into something stronger and more useable to him. You will not become what God wants you to be if you are bitter. It is very easy to become hurt and angry when you are suffering. Ever see a dog in pain? They snarl and can bite. It's a natural reaction. We have to guard against it. Realize that unforgiveness leads to bitterness, which is ugly and destructive. It's like a cancer that selfishly feeds itself and hurts the rest of the body, eventually leading to sickness and death.

The first step is to acknowledge your pain and anger, which isn't sin. It's totally normal for us to experience these emotions. That's how God made us. But what isn't normal is for us to dwell in anger and let it consume us. It's an opportunity for us to trust in God in all things. It's easy to trust Him in the good times but a challenge to do it in bad times.

Give your pain to God in prayer. Lay it down on the altar and let go. That is especially hard to do when someone has intentionally hurt you, but that's when it is most life changing. Take a few minutes to read Psalm 62. David is in a pickle. He is being attacked, and it sure sounds like he is in retreat and without many options. Of God, he says "He is my defense;

I shall not be moved" (verse 6). When we are hurt, we instinctively tend to let our anger rise up, and we use it as a shield of defense. But we need to leave it lying on the ground and pick up God as our shield instead.

David says, "In God is my salvation and my glory; the rock of my strength, and my refuge, is in God. Trust in Him at all times, you people; pour out your heart before Him; God is a refuge for us" (verse 7, 8). Even if your enemies are spewing lies about you in hatred, God is there as your fortress and your refuge. Run into Him for comfort. Once there, you need to give him all your pain and let go of the anger and desire for revenge. Realize that "power belongs to God" (verse 11) and "also to You, O Lord, belongs mercy; For You render to each one according to his work" (verse 12).

There is no way you can fix the wrong that was done to you, so give it up. God's power is infinitely greater than ours, and He will defend you. "Therefore in the shadow of your wings I will rejoice" (Psalm 63:7). He is so much greater than our situation. Under His mighty shadow, we can truly let go of our burdens.

Bear in mind that forgiveness is your key to release and healing. Even when others are clearly hostile toward you and have wronged you, there is sweet relief in surrendering those emotions to God. You don't have to carry them! Let God sweep them away.

It is said that if you don't forgive, you are not having any effect on the person who harmed you. But you will destroy yourself if you hold on to it. When you don't forgive, you are simply feeding the hurt until it grows black in your heart as bitterness. This is exactly what your enemy is trying to do! You can choose to forgive, or you can choose to foster bitterness. It's completely up to you.

Make the decision today to forgive and receive freedom. Say out loud in prayer, "Lord, I forgive (name) for (the hurtful action). I release any bitterness in my heart and trust you to heal my heart completely." After you forgive, simply refuse to entertain further thoughts of hurt and pain. Rebuke the enemy when those feelings or thoughts pop up. Bless that person, out loud if you can, and you will have the victory.

If the person who hurt you is a family member, it may be difficult to avoid further interactions. I strongly recommend you seek counsel from a godly pastor or see a Christian therapist. You don't have to stay friends with someone who hurts you, but you can't easily walk away from family. Wise counsel will help you communicate with that person in a positive way and help you set boundaries for a mutually respectful relationship going forward.

Make the decision today to choose the way of life and healing. Reject bitterness and receive the peace of God which brings true joy! "Teach me your way, O Lord, and lead me in a smooth path, because of my enemies . . . Wait on the Lord; Be of good courage, And He shall strengthen your heart" (Psalm 27:11, 14).

GIVING FORGIVENESS

Lord, I forgive _____________________ for _____________________ .
I release any bitterness in my heart and trust you to heal my heart completely. Amen.

Focus on Strengths and Be Willing to Work on Weaknesses

We all have different personalities, thankfully! I am an introvert, and my husband is an extrovert. He will talk to anyone, anywhere, about anything. I'm very good at organizing, while that is not one of his strengths. He is very creative and good at brainstorming ideas. I'm more of a list person; I enjoy structure and will move down my to-do list methodically.

We know that, often, opposites attract. It seems we intuitively seek out others who have qualities we admire and wish we had. While the adage that your spouse completes you is not biblical, it does represent the truth that we can complement each other and, as a couple, have more skills and abilities than one does alone.

However, our differences can lead to conflict, and, all too often, stress is the instigator-in-chief. Have you ever been under work stress and taken it out on your family members at home? When we are stressed, we have typical coping behaviors. On our own, these behaviors don't hurt anyone else, but they can keep us stuck in our stress. In a family, though, these behaviors can hurt everyone else. This not only keeps us stuck in stress mode, but it intensifies the stress because now you're hurting someone else, and then they get stressed, too.

When we accept our differences, we can use our strengths to help each other. You may be very good at a coping skill that I'm not good at, so we would be stronger together. If we pool our positive coping resources, then as a family, we can overcome and lift each other out of our swamp of self-pity and frustration. When you understand how God made you, you will be more appreciative of Him. You will also see your weaknesses as an opportunity to become more like Him.

I withdraw into myself when I am stressed. I simply don't want to deal with anyone else in any way. After my workday is done, if I have had to deal with patient cases that were difficult, the last thing I want to do is be social. I tend to get irritable. I am not naturally good at communicating my feelings, which leads to my husband feeling rejected or wondering if I'm mad at him. The truth is that it really isn't personal, I just don't like dealing with anyone at that moment and need time by myself to recover. This is an area I have had to work on quite a bit.

However, I am very good at not becoming emotional. I can stoically move through whatever happens without reacting quickly or harshly. I rationally assess the situation, weigh options, make a decision, and then move forward. I don't yell, complain, or get fearful. I don't get stuck in indecision and feel helpless. A lot of this is just who I am, but going to medical school, internship, and residency forces you to do this all day long. Who wants a doctor who falls apart in an emergency, right?

My husband reacts to stress somewhat differently. He can rationally assess an emergency and move forward, but if it's just regular, daily stress, he gets totally off track from what he was working on. He loses focus and gets emotional. It's very difficult for him to put his thoughts and emotions about an issue aside to think about something else. Part of it may be his Hispanic background, but he feels and expresses stress passionately. He also gets frustrated when we don't listen to him when he's stressed and trying to problem solve. He can get very irritable without even being aware of it because he's reacting based on his feelings and a heavy feeling of responsibility. Unlike me, he craves time with the family when he's stressed. But as you might imagine, he's not the most fun to be around when he's upset!

But he is very good at allowing himself to feel these emotions and work through them, instead of letting them stew. He never holds a grudge or any resentment. He readily admits when he's been wrong and will quickly ask for forgiveness, which brings us closer and therefore makes us stronger together. He says that Mexican families will shout and argue but then hug it out and go eat tamales!

Like us, when you are under stress, your personality likely leads you into a typical pattern of behavior. Take some time to think about how you respond to stress, and ask family members or good friends to give their observations. Be ready—it may not be pleasant! But you need to know what you're doing right and what you're doing wrong. Think about it honestly, and write down your own observations. Really think about what you feel when you are stressed, and then what you do, and how it affects you and others. Pray for God to give you understanding.

Once you see how you respond, you can tell clearly what is and isn't working. For the things you do well, keep them up! Consider adding some new strategies that may help with your weaknesses. I have learned that if I'm too upset to really talk about something, I can't just shut up and say that nothing's wrong while stuffing my anger or turning it into resentment. I now can tell my husband that I've had a horrible day and I'm really frustrated. I can let him know that I want to tell him about it but only after I've had about twenty minutes by myself to calm down. That way, he feels loved and not rejected, and he is more than happy to give me the time I need alone to self-regulate. Then when I feel better, we both feel appreciated and are on the same page when discussing the situation.

Other strategies are going for a short walk around the block or taking a short time to go pray and breathe deeply. You may also want to call that accountability partner who can listen to you vent. They can hear your story and then offer honest advice.

If you have habits that are not helping your stress, determine now how you can start to make some changes. In addition to needing alone time after a hard day, I also will admit that I am a workaholic. My sister has called me that since we were kids! This is good if you have a thousand things to do, because you get them done. But this type of work stress can hurt your family. I tend to complete work tasks at the expense of family time. My husband is hurt by this because he feels unimportant and rejected. Not knowing when to quit only increases my work stress, and then it adds to my home stress. I have learned over the years that my inbox will never truly be empty, and tomorrow is another day. And most importantly, family is much more important than work.

Get out your journal and take some time to determine what you're doing well and what you need to work on. Share your commitment with your accountability partner who will help you pray about it. Be willing to change and then do it. Your stress will immediately be much less of a problem!

Accountability Partner

There is a powerful Biblical principle of accountability. Some of us are more self-driven and can motivate ourselves. Some people (like several of my kids, *you guys know who you are!*) struggle for years with not being self-motivated. They need external consequences to motivate them to do things. Two of our kids would have failed pretty much every subject when we tried homeschooling if we hadn't hovered over their shoulder every moment of that miserable year. We gave up, because it just was way too much work to force them to do the work. In contrast, another of our kids was very motivated and did about two years of schoolwork in one year, graduating high school early. We all are very different!

When it comes to spiritual growth, especially when going through difficult circumstances, it really helps to have someone walk alongside you. If you're self-driven, you are probably reading this book because you want to learn all you can about stress, and you want to do everything you can to help get through it with good health. You probably are self-motivated. Even so, get someone on board with you to help support you in your healing. Ecclesiastes tells us, "A threefold cord is not quickly broken" (Ecclesiastes 4:12). Bind yourself with another person and with God, creating that threefold cord. If you are seeing a counselor or getting counseling through your church, that person will certainly hold you accountable. If you are not in counseling, ask a good friend or a relative. Consider asking an older member of your church.

When I was newly married and going to a church that, in retrospect, wasn't a good fit, I became quite depressed. I wasn't happy with our church, but my husband loved it. I felt trapped and confused spiritually. I was being told certain things by my pastor and my husband that I didn't agree with, and then I was told that a good wife was submissive. This was a long time ago, but I remember the emotional pain and confusion very well. I felt trapped, controlled, and alone.

One of my patients at the time helped me more than she will ever know. She is significantly older than me and has been in ministry all her adult life. I met her and her husband when I had the privilege of being their doctor, but we became friends after that. She was such a good mentor to me because she listened and gave me wise counsel when I was so confused. It was so empowering for two reasons. First, she reassured me that my perceptions were true and the things I was doing were right. I needed that perspective because I thought I was going crazy! Second, she cautioned me not to get bitter and angry, which I definitely needed to hear. Instead, she encouraged me in healthy ways of dealing with my problem instead of wallowing in anger and self-pity. Without her, I truly don't think I would have gotten through it without lasting emotional damage.

Whomever you find to be your accountability partner, make sure you are open and honest about the issues you are facing. You do not have to explain every little detail about what you're going through. Avoid the temptation to just dump all your complaints on them, because simply complaining and getting sympathy isn't always helpful. Methodically explain what is happening, how it makes you feel, what you are doing in response, and the results of that response. Together, plan for better choices in your response.

Like I've said before, one of my favorite underrated scriptures is Habakkuk 2:2: "Write the vision and make it plain on tablets, that he may run who reads it." Anytime you have a vision, a dream, or a plan, there is power in writing it down. Just seeing it on paper has creative force and is the first step to it becoming reality. If you need to, break it down into smaller steps. For example, don't say "I will treat my spouse better." Really consider what that means. Do you need to change your tone of voice? What you say? How you roll your eyes? How you mutter something and walk away? Be specific.

We will talk about this more in the chapter on your Strategic Plan, but your accountability partner will help you separate your emotions from what needs to be an intentional behavioral plan. As I write this, my playlist is playing "Bridge over Troubled Water" by Simon and Garfunkel. Although I think God is really the ultimate bridge for us, our brother or sister is often a gift God gives us to help us walk over those turbulent waters and move into the future.

Who can help keep you accountable? Reach out to them. Agree on how you will connect and how often. Will you call, email, video chat, or talk in person? Make a plan and stick to it. Writing down a plan with concrete action steps dramatically increases the likelihood you will do it, and your success is virtually guaranteed.

Study the Word

Paul tells Timothy, "Study to shew thyself approved unto God, a workman that needeth not to be ashamed, rightly dividing the word of truth" (2 Tim 2:15 KJV). In his letter to the Ephesians, he writes, "Above all, taking the shield of faith with which you will be able to quench all the fiery darts of the wicked one. And take the helmet of salvation, and the sword of the Spirit, which is the word of God" (Ephesians 6:16–17).

We can't go any farther until we talk about our greatest offensive weapon—the Word of God. You can eat right, practice deep breathing exercises, and even pray, but unless we pick up our swords, we are only on defense. We need to go on offense against the dark forces of this world. Ephesians 6 lists all the components of the armor of God. The body is covered with God's righteousness, salvation, truth, and the gospel of peace, and the warrior holds the shield of faith, but all of that is defensive weaponry. The one offensive weapon used to inflict injury on the enemy is "the sword of the Spirit, which is the word of God" (Ephesians 6:17). Hebrews further tells us, "For the word of God is living and powerful, and sharper than any two-edged sword, piercing even to the division of soul and spirit" (Hebrews 4:12).

One of the crucial tools you must master to defeat stress is how to use the Word of God. I cannot emphasize how powerful the Word is and how important it is to your victory! If you get nothing else from this book, simply start speaking the promises of the Word of God out loud. Everything else will fall into place, and you will begin to rise above your stress.

There is a reason why Jesus prayed, "Give us this day our daily bread" (Matthew 6:11). He was showing us that we need the Word every day. We recently had a weekly Bible study at church that was a little different than others before. We didn't study one topic, one book, or do any author's Bible study. We simply studied the Bible in general. We all learned how to really dig in and study the Word. We started in the Psalms and then read texts from both the Old and New Testament. We read the chapter or chapters in different versions, we wrote them out by hand, and then we really dug in. We picked our favorite verses, looked at who wrote the texts, and then looked at when and why each passage was written. Then we picked all kinds of amazing nuggets out of the sections. It was interesting to see how different verses impacted us all in different ways.

The Word is living. It is God speaking to you. Depending on your situation, God will use His Word to guide you and encourage you. It's like a shortwave frequency that God is using to talk *personally to you*. You just have to tune in, and reading the Word allows you to do just that. I strongly recommend getting out your journal for your study of the Word and what God is speaking to you. I just pulled out my journal to see what I wrote this time last year. One year ago, I wrote down 1 Peter 5:8. "Be sober, be vigilant, because your adversary the devil walks about like a roaring lion, seeking whom he may devour." I also wrote this: *He is not a lion—he only roars like one.*

This is so true, and I would do better if I remembered this! My enemy may sound dangerous and scary, but the only real lion in this story is the Lion of Judah—*Jesus*. I've heard it preached that the devil is a toothless lion who just roars a lot. While you don't want to fall into a trap of complacency, don't ever forget that you are a child of the King, and you have all the power of the Kingdom available to use against the enemy. One of the most powerful tools is the Word of God. Sharpen your sword by reading the Word and studying it. And get ready to start swinging it.

Speak the Word

The ultimate example of the immense power of the Word was given to us by Jesus. When He went into the wilderness, He was tempted by Satan himself. He was tempted to turn stones into bread and was offered all the kingdoms of the world if He would only worship Satan. Every time

Satan spoke, Jesus rebuked him with the Word, and it worked powerfully. The first time, "It is written again, 'You shall not tempt the Lord your God'" (Matthew 4:7). The next time He said, "It is written again, you shall not tempt the LORD your God" (Matthew 4:7). The last time, he probably shouted: "Away with you, Satan! For it is written, 'You shall worship the Lord your God, and Him only you shall serve'" (Matthew 4:10). Three times He says, "It is written."

There is immense power in speaking the Word of God out loud when you pray. Reading and studying the Word is foundational and encouraging, but we wage war in the spiritual realm with our enemy. Spiritual battles cannot be fought by natural means. We must use the Spirit and the Word to fight in the spiritual realm. When you speak the Word of God out loud, it's like putting a bullet in your weapon and firing it. That weapon may look powerful, but until it is loaded and fired, it's useless. Likewise, your faith and your Christianity look good on the outside, but are not enough to defeat evil spiritual forces. You need to use your faith by speaking the promises of God out loud. Consider this: the Word is in a book you read, and it's in your mind, but when you speak it into the universe, you are using the power it contains and you are directing it to do what it was designed for. There is a creative power in the spiritual realm when the Word of God is spoken. It crashes through spiritual opposition and makes way for goodness and blessing.

Bear in mind that the Word of God is God. The Gospel of John starts off with, "In the beginning was the Word, and the Word was with God, and the Word was God." So the Word is God himself. Verse 3 says "All things were made through Him." Him God or Him the Word? That's a trick question, because they are the same! The Word of God is He who created the entire world. Think about that. The eternal, all-powerful God spoke the world into existence, so the Word created everything you know. That is stunning and should cause you to see how powerful spoken words are in our world.

I have a patient who is a successful life coach for women. Her background is in the field of linguistics, which is the study of language. She is a firm believer that when we intentionally speak what we want to happen, it will happen. Science shows neural pathways that start off rough can become stronger the more they are used.[56] For example, if you grew up with your parent telling you that you are ugly, you will believe it for years afterward. This pathway will be fixed in your brain. However, you can choose to tell yourself that you are beautiful and created by God, and when you continue to repeat that over time, you will start to believe it. We never used to think that neurons were all that changeable, but we were wrong. You absolutely can change your reality by using speech in a positive way.

In the spiritual realm, this is exponentially true because God's power flows through His Word! Start off by simply saying out loud to your-self every day, "I can do all things through Christ who strengthens me" (Philippians 4:13). The more you say it, the more you will believe it. The force of the Spirit will greatly amplify your words of faith, and you will be filled with His strength. I promise you, it works!

Start by reading your Bible or your journal and look for Scriptures that really speak to you. Get yourself some Bible highlighters and start marking up your Bible. Right now I'm looking at the highlighted verse in my Bible from Psalm 3:3: "But You, O LORD, are a shield for me, my glory and the One who lifts up my head." Anytime I feel attacked, I speak this out loud. God is my shield, and, by speaking the Word out loud, His power moves forward in my circumstance and He can defend me. You need to speak the Word into the natural world to see the maximum effect it can have in the natural world.

I have four index cards in my Bible which have been there for the last ten years. When I had my solo family medicine practice in Ohio, I went through several years of severe financial hardship. The business was drowning in debt from start-up expenses, and I was barely making enough to pay expenses, so there was very little left over to pay myself. It was a hard burden to bear, because everyone assumes doctors are rich. My patients were coming to me for help with their problems, so I felt like I had no one I could really talk to who would understand. One year, my family had to use the church food bank. It was a very humbling experience.

One of my favorite patients was a sweet, solid woman of faith. She was always so grateful for me but it was truly my privilege to know her. It came up in conversation one day about the financial struggle I was in, and she gave me several verses handwritten on those index cards. One is, "The blessing of the Lord brings wealth, without painful toil for it" (Proverbs 10:22 NIV). Another one is, "The Lord will cause your enemies who rise against you to be defeated before your face; they shall come out against you one way and flee before you seven ways. The Lord will command the blessing on you in your storehouses and in all to which you set your hand, and he will bless you in the land which the Lord your God is giving you" (Deuteronomy 28:7–8).

I cannot tell you how many times I have said those verses out loud in prayer! You just can't help but feel encouraged when you say those words. But know this: Even if you feel nothing, there is still a powerful force moving through the spoken Word of God. You don't have to feel it for it to be working. The Word is a powerful pathway for God to use to work on your behalf.

Another example of the power of the spoken word is the Aaronic blessing. Warren Marcus wrote the book *The Priestly Prayer of the Blessing* which dives deep into the Aaronic blessing from Numbers 6:22-26.[57] God told Moses to instruct Aaron and his sons exactly how to bless the people.

> *"The LORD bless you and keep you;*
> *The LORD make His face shine upon you,*
> *And be gracious to you;*
> *The LORD lift up His countenance upon you,*
> *And give you peace."*

In Warren's book, he thoroughly explains the meaning of each of these lines. It is stunningly beautiful how much God loves us and wants to bless us. But beyond just appreciating how much good God has for us, we need to look at how it comes about. God told Moses to tell Aaron and his sons that this is how you shall bless the children of Israel. They were clearly told by God to speak the words of the prayer over the people. Could God have blessed the people without these words being spoken? Sure. But as is often the case, God chooses to move through his children. It's more fun that way. It's like helping your child make chocolate chip cookies. While you can make them perfectly well on your own, it's so much more fun to teach your kids how and to enjoy when they do it! When Aaron spoke this blessing over the people, God moved and blessed them, and they became the great nation of Israel. Verse 27 says, "So they shall put My name on the children of Israel, and I will bless them." The first word is "so," meaning, "in this way" or "by doing this." By speaking the blessing, God was able to move on their behalf.

The words we speak have a lot of power, both for good and for evil. James 3:9, 10 says, "With it [the tongue] we bless our God and Father, and with it we curse men, who have been made in the similitude of God. Out of the same mouth proceed blessing and cursing. My brethren, these things ought not to be so." Just as we have the creative power of God in our mouths, we can destroy with words also. We all know how quickly we can hurt someone with words. Many of us don't realize, though, that we are hindering our success by lazy words. It's so easy to express doubt that is cloaked in faith. How can that be?

Have you ever said, "If it's God's will, we will get the house?" or "If it's the Lord's will to heal him" or even "I don't see how I'll pass that test, but maybe God has something else for me." Start listening and you'll hear a lack of faith in your speech. We temper our expressions of faith by giving God an out, thinking we will be faithful sufferers if things don't go the way we want to. It's a form of martyrdom and rejects the Word of God.

That isn't God's will! He calls us to bold faith. Paul prayed, "That I may open my mouth boldly to make known the mystery of the gospel" (Ephesians 6:19). God expects us to be bold and to speak the Word that pertains to what we are believing for. Another of my favorite verses is "For You, O LORD, will bless the righteous; With favor You will surround him as with a shield" (Psalm 5:12). I often say this with a strong emphasis on "will." This is my bold proclamation of faith. I know my God, I know His Word, and I am fully expecting to be blessed! Be bold with your faith, as the writer of Hebrews tells us, "Let us therefore come boldly to the throne of grace, that we may obtain mercy and find grace to help in time of need" (Hebrews 4:16).

When Jesus passed by the fig tree that wasn't bearing figs, he cursed it. Later, when he walked by it with Peter, Peter was surprised: "Rabbi, look! The fig tree that You cursed has withered away" (Mark 11:21). It's rather funny, in fact. Why was Peter surprised? Jesus further emphasizes the power of speaking your faith: "Have faith in God. For assuredly, I say to you, whoever says to this mountain, 'Be removed and be cast into the sea,' and does not doubt in his heart, but believes that those things he says will be done, he will have whatever he says. Therefore I say to you, whatever things you ask when you pray, believe that you receive them, and you will have them" (Mark 11:22–24).

The book of Joshua starts with God commanding Joshua to go forth into Canaan to conquer the land: "No man shall be able to stand before you all the days of your life; as I was with Moses, so I will be with you. I will not leave you nor forsake you" (Joshua 1:5). (This is a great scripture to memorize and say out loud, changing the "you" to "me.") God next tells Joshua to be strong and courageous, and to follow the law, but that's not all.

Verse 8 has the key to the success of the entire nation of Israel conquering the Promised Land: "This Book of the Law shall not depart from your mouth, but you shall meditate in it day and night, that you may observe to do according to all that is written in it. For then you will make your way prosperous, and then you will have good success."

Simply thinking about the Word isn't enough. You need to act on the Word, and it needs to constantly be coming out of your mouth. Why? "Out of the abundance of the heart his mouth speaks" (Luke 6:45). What is in your heart and mind will come out in your speech. When you are speaking the Word consistently, God fills your heart even more, and you become more like Him and more useful to Him and the kingdom. Speaking the Word is a lot more than just a way to have your problems solved. It changes you! It increases your faith. It makes you stronger. It helps you give to others instead of wallowing in self-pity. You become more like Jesus.

Find a few scriptures every week that speak to your circumstance and write them down. Pray them out loud. Speak them boldly and watch God move!

Speak Your Faith

Take a moment to really understand how much power we have with our speech. We just discussed how we can bless others and bless situations by speaking the Word of God. But it goes even beyond the Word. We are called to speak our faith into circumstances. Our voice should proclaim God's Word, but when we connect to it to our faith, we immediately have access to His power.

What is faith? It is agreeing with God. You may not realize that when we speak faith, we are creating a pathway for God to move in. When you have unbelief or simply don't speak faith, the Spirit is hindered and simply cannot do much for you. There is a blockage in the spiritual realm. You can stop the blessing God is trying to send to you by the words you say. Jesus tells us in Matthew, "A good man out of the good treasure of his heart brings forth good things, and an evil man out of the evil treasure brings forth evil things. But I say to you that for every idle word men may speak, they will give account of it in the day of judgment. For by your words you will be justified, and by your words you will be condemned" (Matthew 12:35–37).

Our words are powerful! Even words that just slip out—*thoughtless words*—can create a reality we do not want. We need to remove these from our speech. Think about what encouragement feels like. When you get a pep talk from a friend, their words imprint on your spirit and give you fresh power, lifting your mood.

Remember that the Creator of the universe lives within you! Imagine the Spirit of God hovering over the waters in the beginning. There was nothing, but within six days, there was the entire world. God created the land, the sun, and all the animals simply by speaking. Likewise, there is immense creative power in speaking your faith.

As believers we are composed of body, soul (mind), and spirit (God's Spirit). When you speak doubt from your soul, it suppresses the Spirit.

But when you allow the powerful Spirit of God that lives within you to speak boldly, positively, and in faith, God moves.

This is such a powerful and crucial concept, and I struggled with this for a long time. As a perfectionist, I tend to see the things that aren't right, and I don't always hold back my criticism. When my mood gets low, I tend to complain. But I have realized that God can't easily fix things when I am negative and critical, because my faith is low. I imagine God leaning against the wall with his arms folded, just quietly watching me with a small smile on his face. He's patiently waiting and saying, *"Let me know when you're done being negative. I have all day."* Have you ever put your toddler into time out until he or she calmed down? God steps out of our way when we are negative and is just waiting for us to give up and embrace His way.

I can't say that I have this perfected yet. But I have gotten a lot better at not saying anything negative and instead declaring what I am believing for. The saying, "You get what you pay for" is more aptly phrased, "You get what you declare for."

In Matthew 16, Jesus gave Peter the keys to heaven. Jesus told him, "Whatever you bind on earth will be bound in heaven, and whatever you loose on earth will be loosed in heaven" (verse 19). But if you read starting in verse 13, you will see that this is all about their speech. Jesus asked, "Who do men say that I, the Son of Man, am?" The answer was, "Some say John the Baptist, some Elijah, and others Jeremiah or one of the prophets" (verse 14). Jesus then asks, "But who do you say that I am?" Simon then says, "You are the Christ, the Son of the living God." Jesus says, "I say to you that you are Peter, and on this rock I will build My church, and the gates of Hades shall not prevail against it" (verse 15–18).

Simon's name changed because he not only received the revelation of who Jesus was, but he spoke it out loud. Then Jesus spoke the blessing into Peter's life. This power wasn't just for Peter, but also for us. Whatever we bind or loose on earth will happen due to our words. If we bind the enemy with the Word of God, he is bound. If we loose blessings into our lives with our words of faith, the power of God will release them. The keys are our words, because they can unlock the heavens!

When we speak our faith, we are declaring to the world (and the enemy) that we know God is willing and able to fix everything that is wrong. When our faith is spoken out loud, it opens a path in the spiritual realm that the Spirit moves into very easily, and it will sweep us toward an answer. But when we speak doubt and fear, we are closing off that path, blocking the movement of the Spirit.

Consider all the examples in the book of Acts where the apostles spoke boldly and God moved. They sang praises in prison and the doors miraculously unlocked. The lame were healed. They boldly preached the gospel to the Sanhedrin. They continued to preach after being specifically "commanded not to speak at all nor teach in the name of Jesus" (Acts 4:18). Their answer? "For we cannot but speak the things which we have seen and heard" (Act 4:20). Not long after, they prayed for even more boldness: "Now Lord, look on their threats, and grant to Your servants that with all boldness they may speak Your word" (Acts 4:29). Tabitha was raised from the dead after Peter prayed for her. Peter even went to Cornelius and preached the gospel to the Gentiles, which was really bold! These miracles were brought about by the apostles speaking forth with power and with faith.

Before skeptics start saying, *"Here we go, name it and claim it"*, I am not talking about selfish accumulation. The rich man obviously had a lot of wealth, but he was tormented in hell. Similarly, the rich young ruler was unwilling to give of his possessions to follow Jesus. If you're just looking to store up wealth and possessions for yourself and you are unwilling to use it for the Kingdom, the words of faith you speak will not be in alignment with the Will of God, so the anointing power of the Spirit will not make you rich.

This principle of spoken faith depends on your motives. If you are believing for a new car or a boat, but you are only wanting it for selfish reasons, God won't necessarily bless that. When you want something that doesn't line up with God's will for you, it usually doesn't work out. However, if your car is old and unreliable, which affects your ability to get to church or fellowship with others, go ahead and believe God for a new one. There is nothing at all wrong with expecting a harvest on the seed you sow into the kingdom. This includes financial seed and harvest. But if your motivation for financial increase is purely selfish, God can't honor that. One of my favorite sayings is, "Our motivation for accumulation is distribution." If you had enough money in the bank as an emergency fund and enough so that you only had to work as much as you really wanted to, what could you do with your time? What if you were wealthy and could retire? Would you be able to volunteer in ministry more? Give more? Do more for others? Wealth is not evil. Money is simply a tool that can be used for good. If you are believing God for more resources so that you can give more and do more in the kingdom, God will honor that and bless you.

If you find yourself in a tough situation, don't simply accept it. While God does minister to us in poverty or in sickness, or even in death, there is nothing wrong with using your faith for something better. In fact, God expects us to!

Many Christians under appreciate how much power we do have with our faith and our words. If God created the world in six days by speaking it forth, don't you see how we can access that power and speak things into our lives? God loves to give good gifts to us, but sadly, we often don't even ask or we don't ask in faith. Remember that when you speak doubt, you are empowering the enemy's forces. You are fueling the negative power at work. Don't do that! Give power to the work of the Spirit.

But what if you don't see results? Realize that there is difference between your responsibility and God's. Your part is to be full of faith and boldly speak the results you are believing for. God's part is whether and how He does it. If you haven't yet seen the results you want, keep standing strong and believing: "Having done all, to stand" (Ephesians 6:13). But if you don't speak words of faith, then it's your fault if you don't get what you want. You closed the door.

Sometimes this process takes time, which the enemy uses to try to discourage you. Don't let him! Hold fast in faith. Sometimes the delay is because God is waiting on you to do something. Then it will be His turn to do something. It may take some prayer and discernment to know if it's your turn or His turn. But when it's God's turn, learn to wait on Him and believe. Kenneth Copeland says when you are in between "Amen" and "Hallelujah," you simply stand in faith for as long as it takes to receive your answer. It might take a while, but after you've prayed, "Watch, stand fast in the faith, be brave, be strong" (I Corinthians 16:13).

The psychology community has looked at the relationship between positive affirmations and depression and anxiety. Anxiety is experiencing intrusive thoughts that create worry or fear, whether they have any validity or basis in reality. Perspective is often lost when anxiety creates worry. A study showed that replacing anxious thoughts with either positive images or positive verbal affirmations showed a decrease in worrisome thoughts.[58] Another study in patients with a chronic disease (chronic stress) showed that self-affirmation correlated to a decrease in depression.[59] This study used the strategies of putting things in perspective and reflection on personal values. When you look at your situation with a God perspective, it's much easier to have a better mood and more peace.

Try this out for the next two weeks. Every day, determine to not speak anything that expresses doubt or fear. Reframe all your communication in the context of God's power and His willingness to bless us. Speak your dreams out as if they already are. Say "when" not "if." Say "It's going to be so great when . . ." or "I can't wait until . . ." Even if you don't get everything you speak right away, I promise that your faith will increase. The prayers that do get answered will be sweet and will fill you with joy and even more faith. Then you will be better able to minister to others and you will be more successful in life. If you don't know Toby Mac's song "Speak Life," go look it up on YouTube right now. The lyrics encourage you to speak life into the darkest times of life.

Change in Small, Easy Steps

Spiritually, are there other things you should be doing, but aren't? If you aren't yet fully reborn with salvation through faith in Jesus, find a church and receive salvation! It is freely offered to you through repentance and faith in Jesus. I am sure there is a church near you that will welcome you with open arms and walk with you in your journey.

If you are a Christian, are you attending church regularly, or do you often skip it for less than good reasons? Are you involved with your church family or do you just show up and slip out on Sunday mornings? Do you ever listen to Christian music? As one Christian radio station advertises, "encouraging and uplifting" music can make a big difference in your thoughts and attitudes. What are you spending your time on? Watching sports or reality shows? There are a lot of things that can entertain you, but don't necessarily feed your soul. They aren't inherently wrong, but can be bad for you. Do you watch the NFL network during the week, then watch football all day long Sunday? Football can be a lot of fun, but if it becomes an obsession or more important to you than the people around you, it has become an idol. How about social media? The younger generations are absolutely consumed by social media and virtual social connections, not to mention video games. These things can be an occasional source of entertainment or can become your god and consume all your time and energy.

Many activities will stunt your spiritual power. Some things are permissible (not sinful) but they inhibit your growth. For example, consider nutrition. It's not bad to eat ice cream on occasion. But if you crave it and eat it in large amounts every day instead of fruits and vegetables, you're going to get sick. Now think about your time. Are you intentional and purposeful in the way you spend your time each day? Invest time in prayer, connecting with your family, working your job, ministering to those around you, and building personal skills. Make sure you don't spend too much time on things that don't help you become a better person. Keep perspective and balance in all things, and keep God at the center of what you do.

If you've never seen the movie *What About Bob?* with Bill Murray and Richard Dreyfuss, watch it. It is one of my favorites that puts me in stitches with laughter every time. It's about Bob (Murray), a neurotic New Yorker who sees Dr. Marvin (Dreyfuss), a psychiatrist, for help with his phobias. Dr. Marvin has published a book called *Baby Steps*, which Bob tries to follow. He makes small changes pushing himself out of his comfort zone. This would be a good thing, but Bob follows Dr. Marvin to his New Hampshire lake house on vacation and progressively drives Dr. Marvin absolutely crazy. The patient gets better, and the doctor goes nuts!

Aside from the humor, baby steps are the key concept here. If you have a teenager skipping school and in legal trouble, you are going to be angry. But separating your emotions from the reality is a baby step. Letting go of the things you have no control over is another step. Changing your response to his poor choices is another step.

The old saying is very true, "The best way to eat an elephant is one bite at a time." No one overcomes overnight, especially when you have been wronged or suffered great loss. But you cannot be stagnant and paralyzed by inaction. No matter where you are, make sure you are always improving and moving forward. Baby steps will keep you moving in the right direction.

Perfectly Imperfect

I had a patient tell me the other day that she was addicted to the false sense of control. I have been thinking about it ever since, because I also love when I feel in control. Control makes you feel powerful and gives you a sense of security. When you're out of control (skidding down an icy road), you immediately are terrified of what might happen. When I meticulously make a to-do list for a Saturday, and then I check off everything by 2 p.m., I feel amazing! I have a hard time writing or relaxing if there are still things on my to-do list. My younger sister and I are a year and a half apart in age. She used to get mad at me for a lot of things, deservedly so. One was that I was a perfectionist. She made fun of me not only for making my bed in the morning, but for making sure it was neatly made before I climbed in at night. If the covers were askew and not tucked in right when I went to bed, it didn't feel right and would drive me nuts. I had to make it perfect before climbing in. (Yes, I'm the one with OCD tendencies, and she's the normal one!)

As an adult, I relax when I control my home. When all the clutter is put away and my home has a zen-like peace (I can hear you laughing . . . *you know it rarely happens!*) I can relax. But life gets in the way! I don't have a *Better Homes and Gardens* home. My living room is unlikely to be featured in *Good Housekeeping*. I have had to learn a difficult truth—we are never really in control and it's all an illusion.

If your kitchen is remodeled and sparkling clean with a platter of cupcakes and fresh flowers on it, you feel like you have no problems. But you could have a cancer in your brain that don't know about. If your workday goes smoothly and you clean out your email inbox by 4:55 p.m. and walk out on time, you feel like a success. But your brother may have just had a car accident. No matter how good you feel about your accomplishments or your environment, you are not really in control. That's exactly why we all need God.

We need to remind ourselves that any feeling of control we have is temporary at best and untrue at worst. I like to say that we have faith for the express purpose of using it. Exercise your faith. Quit thinking you have to know everything and control everything. *Let go and let God*, as the saying goes. It is so freeing to completely and utterly trust God.

For non-believers, all you have is yourself. Your work, your accomplishments, your thoughts. You have nothing beyond that. When troubles come, your foundation is like sand. You may sink in despair. But when a Christian endures the stormy winds, his house is built on the rock. The winds and rain still belt the house, but it stays firmly attached to the rock and doesn't budge. The Christian knows the rain will end and he will still have the rock. He isn't surprised by the rain. That's exactly why he built his house on the rock!

Don't be surprised when stress and trials hit you. Job went through the worst of the worst, but he never gave up his faith in God. If it's a season of sunshine for you now, be grateful for it and don't be surprised if it doesn't last forever.

If your personality is like mine and you like things neat and orderly, learn to live with some degree of mess in your life. Let your closet get messy, or let your clothes lay on the bedroom floor once in a while. Let the dishes stack up in the sink overnight so you can watch a movie, then wash them the next day. The more you learn to be comfortable with imperfection, the less stress you will feel. Much of the stress I have had in my life is when things just aren't right. I think that kitchens should be cleaned up after supper and houses should be cleaned every Saturday. In family medicine, I was taught that all patient calls and concerns were addressed before you went home at night. But often, these things can wait until the next day.

I like to think of living for God as "imperfectly perfect." Perfection is when something is of the highest excellence, without flaw or fault. But life in this world is never flawless because of sin. Man is sinful by nature and thus never perfect. God is perfection. Jesus was without sin, flaw, or fault. This is the essence of Christianity: God came to earth as Jesus, a sinless, perfect man, to lay down His life in payment for our sins. God has brought perfection down to be accessed by imperfect man. Perfection came to live in imperfection.

The perfect Spirit resides in our imperfect bodies in an imperfect world.

John the Baptist recognized that Jesus was the Messiah and told his followers just that. He said, "He must increase, but I must decrease" (John 3:30). Jesus must increase in me and in what I do (His perfection), while what I do (my imperfection) will decrease. Think of our imperfection as a word written in dull gray pencil. God's perfection writes directly over the letters with a vibrant colored ink. The letters are the same, and the gray is still there, but it now is beautiful with perfection overshadowing the imperfection.

God welcomes imperfection in our lives, because He wants the glory. When someone accomplishes great things but is arrogant and selfish, God can't use them. But if you realize and accept your imperfections, a humble spirit is something God can use mightily. Moses sure didn't think he was anywhere near good enough to lead the Israelites. He wasn't perfect, that's for sure. But God used him mightily!

When God called Gideon, the Israelites were living under the oppression of the Midianites. The angel of the Lord came to Gideon and said, "The LORD is with you, you mighty man of valor" (Judges 6:12). I can imagine Gideon looking around, saying, "Who, me?" Like Moses, he thought God was making a mistake in choosing him. The angel tells him, "'Go in this might of yours, and you shall save Israel from the hand of the Midianites. Have I not sent you?' So he said to Him, 'O my Lord, how can I save Israel? Indeed my clan is the weakest in Manasseh, and I am the least in my father's house'" (Judges 6:14–15).

After God winnowed Gideon's men down to a mere three hundred, God gave him a great victory over the enemy. God had to make sure it was obvious to everyone that they didn't do it on their own, but it was a miracle of God. This is how perfection works through our imperfection. Gideon realized that, and afterwards, he refused to take any glory. "Then the men of Israel said to Gideon, 'Rule over us, both you and your son, and your grandson also: for you have delivered us from the hand of Midian.' But Gideon said to them, 'I will not rule over you, nor shall my son rule over you; the LORD shall rule over you'" (Judges 8:22–23).

When we allow God to use us through the messy parts of life, His perfection works a wonderful work in us and others. Hearts are changed and His love flows through people. God gets the glory, not us. God loves using people who know they are imperfect. They don't steal any glory from God. Be imperfectly perfect! When it comes to God, *just okay* is all He asks for. There is no way we can ever be good enough or do enough to *earn* His love. We cannot earn salvation or blessing. We need to bring our mediocrity and even our failures to Him . . . that's where He can really work.

I love the lyrics to the song "Maybe It's Ok" by We Are Messengers. The lyrics point out all the good that can happen after pain, loss, and failure. Heartbreak is the studio where God the Artist goes to work and paints a beautiful masterpiece with all the colors of our pain and grief. Take time to listen to this song and remind yourself of the One who is holding your life together.

Faith Puts God on the Throne

The whole purpose of faith in God is to trust Him and let go. You simply cannot trust in your own sense of control. Faith often is inversely related to your sense of control. When you feel like you have it all handled, you rely on God less. When you know you aren't in control, you reach out to Him in your need. Stress can push us in the wrong way if we aren't careful.

When you are stressed about your situation and thinking anxiously about it all the time, you are not trusting God. When your father was driving your family to an outing growing up, were you anxiously watching his every move? Were you worried he would put his foot on the right pedal, go the right way, and use all the gizmos on the dashboard correctly? No! You probably were getting into trouble with your siblings in the back seat. You trusted that your dad knew how to drive a car, he knew the way, and you were going to arrive safely. Do you ever doubt that the light switch will turn on the light or the handle on the faucet will let the water come out? You just have faith those things will happen.

I remember the story of the old woman who lived in a small town in the central plains where storms and tornadoes are common. She got up every morning and prayed at dawn, sitting on her rocking chair on the porch. One day, a tornado was coming. She was sitting on the porch in her rocking chair, watching the approaching storm. The people in the town were all frantic, looking for shelter, and praying for help. One of them asked her why she wasn't panicking like everyone else and why she wasn't praying. She simply replied, "Unlike you, I done my prayin' this morning, and it's all going to be just fine." Imagine that kind of faith!

Faith in God is letting go of worry about the things He is totally in control of. And He is in control. Even when everything seems to be going wrong. Consider Job. Was God still in control when Job lost his sons and daughters, or when he broke out in sores all over? You bet. When tragedy strikes and we lose a loved one, God is still in control. When you lose your job and run out of money, God is still in control. You just have to believe that. Even when you don't see the answer. For this moment, this minute, this hour, this day, just believe. Walk out on the water. You won't sink in despair . . . your spirit will keep you going and see you through.

Take a minute to listen to Jason Gray's song "I'm Gonna Let It Go." I love this song because he describes what anxiety is like in real terms. The heart of the song is, "Cause if I trusted, I could move with your flow."

Faith Makes a Path for the Spirit to Move and Do Amazing Things

Trusting God and letting Him use us as we go through stress and afterward is a strong testimony to others. God truly does want you to get through it and come out on the other side stronger and increased in faith. Your witness can work powerful things.

Nick Vujicic is an amazing man. He is an inspirational speaker who has overcome quite a bit of handicap. He is happy, energetic, and full of faith, and he makes everyone else's problems seem petty. God uses him mightily. What is his disability? He was born without arms or legs! Check him out online and listen to some of his speeches. In the past, he had some low times of depression. It was just so easy for him to think, "What's the point? What good am I to anyone with everything I cannot do?" But he persevered, and now his speeches and books have reached millions. He is truly inspirational.

Another one of my heroes was Byron Sellers, the children's ministry pastor at our church in Charlotte. Although he graduated to Heaven a few years ago, he had a profound effect on all who had the privilege of knowing him. Despite an enormous disability, and actually because of it, he had a special ministry. Byron was the special needs pastor at our church, so we met him the first time we visited. He welcomed us and especially welcomed Daniel. We were surprised to see that this pastor of special needs had his own special needs—he was a quadriplegic in an electric wheelchair! He had an accident as a teenager that caused a spinal cord injury, so he had no use of his legs and only partial use of his arms. But he had full use of his spirit and his brain, let me tell you!

He was instrumental in developing a Sunday school class for kids with different abilities. For the first time ever, Daniel had a class to attend Sunday mornings where the staff worked with his abilities and disabilities and did much more than just keeping him happy in a room until church was over. Many other children and their families benefitted from this class. Byron's leadership was a true gift to the church and to many families.

His story is inspiring. He suffered greatly in the physical realm, but he always told the story of how he had a choice to make after his injury. It was a process, but he worked through a lot of depression and anger and then decided to accept God's calling, in whatever fashion it was. God blessed him with an amazing wife, wonderful children, a growing ministry, and a huge church family that all loved him. That's the result of trusting that God is sufficient.

Here is my favorite scripture in the whole Bible: "And God is able to make **all** grace **abound** toward you; that ye, **always** having **all** sufficiency in **all** things, may **abound** to **every** good work" (2 Corinthians 9:8 KJV, emphasis mine). Yes, that verse is positive. But here is the hidden gem: there are seven superlatives in it (*and seven is the number of God's perfection*). Not just some grace, not just adequacy in some things, and we aren't supposed to just do something kind of good once in a while. Read it over and over, emphasizing and meditating on each one of them.

God will help you get through your stress and your struggles. There is victory ahead!

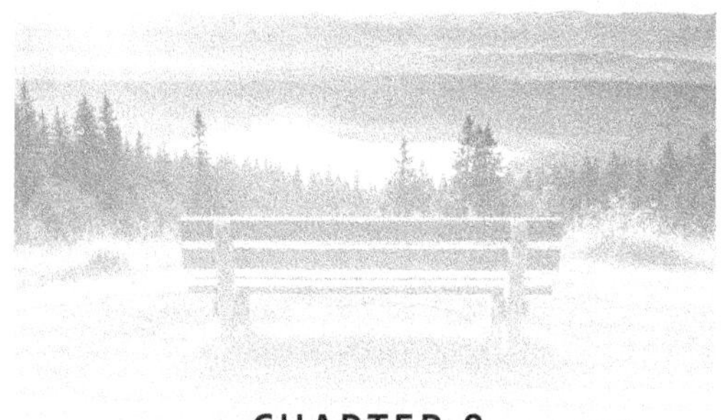

CHAPTER 8

Strategic Plan

Identify your Stress

Now that you know all about stress, it's time to do something about it. Like they say, the definition of insanity is doing the same thing over and over and expecting different results. Instead of just putting the book aside and thinking, "I need to do better," let's actually do something! Let's make an action plan.

The first thing you need to do is set aside time for this planning. This will work best when you dedicate about an hour. Go to a park on a nice day or just get by yourself in the evening. Try to pick a time when you will not be interrupted.

Get out paper and a pen. I know many of you use your laptops and tablets for everything, but I am old school. Research has shown that when you write things down on paper with ink, you learn the information better than just tapping away on a keyboard. You might find that using a pen helps your creative process. But once you are done, feel free to type it up so it looks nice!

Start by writing down all your stresses. Don't worry about whether they are big or small. Just make a nice big list of everything you can think of that causes you stress. If you like, you can use a different page for each major category of stress.

Here's an example of three main areas of stress:

WORK:

> » My supervisor expects more of me than I have time to do.

> » I often work through lunch to stay on top of the work.

> » Co-worker doesn't work as hard as I do, which isn't fair.

> » I haven't had a raise in a long time.

SON:

> » He's getting poor grades now that he's in ninth grade, and he doesn't seem to care.

> » He won't get up in the morning until I yell, and then we all run late.

> » He is constantly on his phone and doesn't want to participate in family activities.

WEIGHT:

> » I need to lose thirty pounds.

> » I am not working out because I don't get home until 6:00 p.m., and then I need to cook dinner.

> » I eat out too much for lunch.

> » I stress eat sweets.

> » I feel ugly and like a failure.

This first step can be therapeutic. Just like journaling, getting those stresses out of your head and onto paper helps that whirling tornado of thoughts and emotions in your brain settle down, and you will start to feel better because you are being honest with yourself.

LIST OUT YOUR STRESSORS

Assess the Effect of Stress

The next step is to write down all the effects you are experiencing from your stressors. Divide them into four categories, like this:

1. Emotional Effects

Do you struggle with anger, fear, disappointment, rejection, unmet expectations?

Honestly think about how you feel when dealing with each of these stresses. Take some time to dig a little deeper. For example, anger is a common reaction to stress. But quite often, anger is the result of fear. For example, if you are mad at your son for getting bad grades, it's usually because you're afraid he's going to be an academic failure and then fail at a career and life in general. That also ties into pride and shame, because if your child turns out to be a totally messed up adult, you feel ashamed as if it must be your fault.

Anger also is often from disappointment and taking things as a personal insult. As parents, we love it when our kids say, "you were right!" or "that was a good idea!" But when they reject our advice or ideas, we feel personally rejected. Everyone who has parented teenagers has learned to not take their rejection personally

Unmet expectations happen all the time when it comes to other people, whether they are family, friend, or co-worker. Sometimes we feel disbelief, pain, embarrassment, frustration, rejection, or even hot-blooded anger. This is the time to be fully honest with yourself and write down everything you feel. Remember, emotions are part of being a human being, and God made us to experience a wide variety of emotions. The Psalms are filled with David's emotions . . . the good, the bad, and the ugly. It's not a sin to feel an emotion. Once you are aware of your feelings, you can make good decisions about how to move forward. So be honest with yourself.

2. Cognitive Effects

Consider how you have reacted to those emotions. Do you suppress them and try to just move on? Do you let it get in your head and dominate your thoughts? Do the emotions affect your job performance or your relationships?

Our reaction to emotions will determine our thoughts. This is where the intentionality of response comes in and where you have all the power. Because in the heat of the moment, we often let our thoughts go where they shouldn't, and we think thoughts that are not productive.

» Do you think hopeless thoughts?

» Do you ruminate about how to fix the other person?

» Do you have a hard time not thinking about work issues at home in the evening?

» Do you get overwhelmed and then lose focus and efficiency?

» Do you withdraw from communicating with someone?

» Do you give up on a task because it's too hard?

Emotions always lead to thoughts, and then, eventually, thoughts either reinforce that emotion or change it to something else. Re-read the section on speaking faith and speaking positively. When you realize that your thoughts are not helping your situation, you are ready to start changing them intentionally.

3. Physical Effects

Write down all the physical symptoms you have been experiencing. If you're like me, you may minimize them and not consider them as significant. But you might be surprised how they can add up. Here are some common symptoms that are associated with stress:

» Fatigue

» Poor sleep

» Neurologic: headaches, numbness or tingling, dizziness

» Mental health: anxiety, depression, apathy, irritability

- » Cognitive: poor memory, poor focus and task completion, perseveration, brain fog
- » Gastrointestinal: indigestion, bloating, changes in bowel movements
- » Hormonal: irregular periods, PMS, low sex drive, erectile dysfunction, menopausal symptoms
- » Cardiac: palpitations, fast heart rate
- » Weight gain

4. Spiritual Effects

The last step is to assess how your stress responses have affected you spiritually. This may be a little hard to admit. Has your stress drawn you closer to God, or have you let yourself drift away? Stress is always an opportunity to draw closer to Him. We know this, but yes, we hate how it feels. But a life devoid of stress and devoid of God is not worth living. We realize that when we come through a storm and feel stronger and closer to God on the other side. It's worth it.

EMOTIONAL EFFECTS

PHYSICAL EFFECTS

COGNITIVE EFFECTS

SPIRITUAL EFFECTS

Before you move on, take a few minutes to pray over these lists. Repent of anything God convicts you of, but mostly just give it all to God and ask Him to walk with you in a new stage of growth to overcome.

Now assess how much of your stress you have control over. Sort your stresses into two categories: those that you have no control over at all, and those that you have some control over.

For example:

NO CONTROL	SOME OR A LOT OF CONTROL
» Dog who barks at everything	» Too tired to get up after staying up late
» Overbearing mother-in-law	» Arguing with child repeatedly
» Teenager getting low grades	» Being overweight
» Cold winter weather	» Marital conflict
» Job layoff	» Overspending
» Medical bills	» Stressful job
» Car needing repairs	» Too busy

You can rewrite the list as two columns, or you can highlight items in two different colors. Once you know what is within your control, you can plan your response. Remember, you can't change what happens to or around you. But you are in control of your response to it.

Also, you may want to sort them by how important it really is in the grand scheme of life. For example, is being ten pounds overweight as important as marital conflict? Is the animal who needs insulin injections twice a day worth your frustration and stress when your children love their pet and get joy from him? Some stresses really aren't worth such an intense reaction. If you were diagnosed with cancer today, would you worry about some of these things? You would probably realize that some of the things might not be as big of a deal as you think they are.

NO CONTROL	SOME OR A LOT OF CONTROL

Make a Detailed Written Plan for Change.

This is the hardest part, and it will take some time. Don't try to do this in ten minutes. I recommend dedicating a few days up to a week to this process. Consider what concrete things you can do to change your stress response. For example, you can get to bed earlier every night so you get a full night's sleep. You can dedicate time in your day for prayer, taking a hot bath, or an exercise class. You can listen to relaxing music in the car instead of the news.

Some changes that seem easy for others will be hard for you! It would be easy for me to tell you to get up at six in the morning every day, because I do it, so it feels like no big deal to me. But for you, that might be very difficult. You might have no problem at all working out at the gym every day at six in the evening, while that would be hard for me because of my schedule and obligations. Write down any ideas or goals you might have, big or small. Pray about them and take some time to really think about it.

If you can't commit to doing something every day (like a spin class or taking a relaxing bath), try committing to doing it once a week. Consider asking someone else to give you advice on ways you can slow down or take more time for you, or other ways you can reduce stress. Having an outside person's perspective can be really enlightening, especially a spouse or trusted friend. Make your action plan as simple or as detailed as you want, but I suggest starting with five to ten changes you can easily make. These can be physical, mental, or spiritual, and the best approach is to have some of each. Write them down, and try to make a related concrete goal.

For any of you whose children have individual education plans (IEPs), you are very familiar with academic goals for children with special needs. Daniel's goal for the year may involve reading comprehension. The goal will be something concrete like, "Daniel will read a short story and answer comprehension questions with 80% accuracy on four out of five trials." With a concrete goal, progress is very measurable.

If your goal is for exercise, a concrete goal might be: "I will ride my bike for thirty minutes, three days per week." When you set a goal, please do not feel like you are a failure for not doing it. It's just a goal, a target of where you are aimed. Underneath your goal, put a bunch of lines and then every week, assess your progress. If you ride your bike thirty minutes only one or two days, that's just fine. Write it down with pride! Over time, you will become more comfortable with your new habit, and you will do it more easily and with joy. Eventually, you can reassess your progress monthly instead of weekly.

IDEAS & GOALS

Yesterday I was trying to work on the budget and pay bills. I had to move money around in various accounts to get everything paid, and it was complicated. I also was trying to pack for a trip. I was trying to get all this done by five o'clock, so I could relax in the evening. None of my account logins were working and before I knew it, I was madder than a hornet! I kept getting interrupted. Soon it was nearly seven o'clock, I still had to pack, and I was hungry and grumpy. I realized how stressed I was, so I quit everything and went out to walk the dog. The fresh air and the fading light was so refreshing, especially with my adorable yellow lab who is so much fun. I came in and was able to get everything done calmly in about thirty minutes. My son and husband were thankful, too.

Have a self-care list ready to deploy as part of your arsenal of weapons when stress goes up. Write a plan for when you inevitably find yourself stressed. For me, one that always works is taking a walk outside. For you it may be taking a bath, playing a video game, or baking a dessert. Whatever it is, have it written down and let your family know so they can understand your needs and can help encourage you to pull your list out and implement it. Just be sure you don't eat that cheesecake all by yourself when you are done baking it!

SELF-CARE LIST

Most importantly, don't forget one of the most powerful weapons when the arrows fly: the Word of God. Find several Scriptures that really speak to you. Write them down on index cards or make a desktop wallpaper of them so they are handy when you need them. Remember: The spoken "word of God is living and powerful, and sharper than any two-edged sword" (Hebrews 4:12), and it will do amazing things when you are stressed. Speaking His Word immediately brings the Spirit into our hearts and minds to bring clarity and peace. Have your weapons of the Word ready for when you need them. Use the defensive weapons used in Ephesians, especially the shield of faith, but when you really want to go on the offensive against your spiritual enemy, get out the sword of the Spirit. The Word used in faith can conquer every effect of stress!

FAVORITE SCRIPTURES

Set Future Dream Goals

Remember, "where there is no vision, the people perish" (Proverbs 29:18 KJV). This is the fun part. You need to dream! After all, one of the goals of turning stress into blessing is to enhance your life and your future. God has great plans for all of us which is one of the main reasons our enemy throws obstacles in our path. Stress can drive us away from God and away from the blessings He has for us. My hope for you is certainly that you analyze your stress to understand it more and to learn how to deal with it more productively, but also that you reach your full potential in Christ. "'For I know the plans I have for you', declares the LORD, 'plans to prosper you and not to harm you, plans to give you hope and a future'" (Jeremiah 29:11 NIV)

I have never been a New Year's resolution gal, but in the past few years, I have taken time every January to review my life goals from the last year and revise them as needed. I have goals regarding my health, my home, my ministry, my finances, and my career. Take a minute to just meditate on the fact that God loves you as much as anyone else on earth. You are His beloved, and He wants to bless you more abundantly than you can ever imagine.

In my practice, I often challenge mid-life folks to consider how healthy they want to be at seventy and eighty. There is no doubt that what you do in your fifties and sixties makes a huge difference in how healthy you will be twenty years down the road. You could be dead, or you could be living a vibrant life with regular exercise, ministry, and social connections. But you have to invest in yourself to get the desire outcome.

Your goals should include career goals, family life goals, emotional goals, and spiritual or ministry goals. They can be expansive, like "start a non-profit working with the homeless" or more specific like "family game night every Friday." For financial goals, most experts recommend having three to six months of expenses in emergency savings. Set a goal to save a little money every month, and you can get it done. That is true with any goal. Remember baby steps? It all starts with envisioning your dream and then taking those small steps.

Write a paragraph of what your life would look like without stress. It may seem silly and sound ridiculous, but it might help you realize that it's a goal to aim for. What if only half of that vision came true? Wouldn't that be amazing? Dream big and go for it!

Pray and watch God work. When we speak our faith and speak the Word, God has room to work. Don't close the door to the Spirit's move by your speech. "Ye have not, because ye ask not" (James 4:2 KJV). Don't lose out on a blessing just because you didn't ask! God often has the answer just waiting for us, but He patiently waits for us to ask. This is easy. "Ask, and it will be given to you; seek, and you will find; knock, and it will be opened to you. For everyone who asks receives, and he who seeks finds, and to him who knocks it will be opened" (Matthew 7:7–8).

Believe in the promises of God. You are part of the covenant God made with Abraham, and He wants to pour blessings into your life. "Have faith in God. For assuredly, I say to you, whoever says to this mountain, 'Be removed and be cast into the sea,' and does not doubt in his heart, but believes that those things he says will be done, he will have whatever he says. Therefore I say to you, whatever things you ask when you pray, believe that you receive them, and you will have them" (Mark 11:22–24).

God wants you to enter the promised land, inhabit it, and thoroughly enjoy the milk and honey. But you need to step out in faith and do the work to get there. It's worth it! "Eye has not seen, nor ear heard, nor have entered into the heart of man the things which God has prepared for those who love Him" (I Corinthians 2:9).

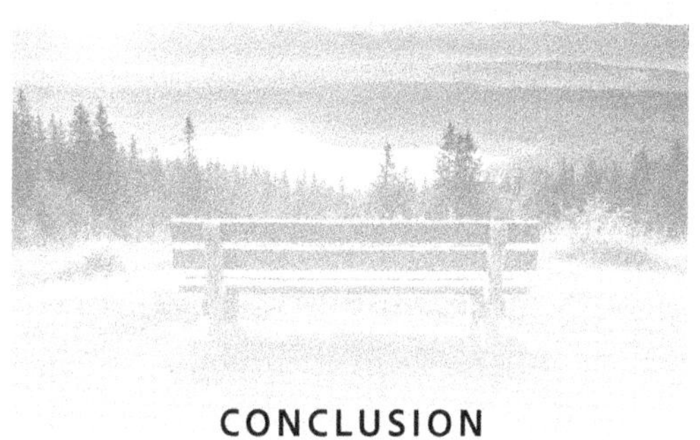

Fully Blessed

Your challenge now, my friend, is to choose your path forward into God's best for you. I can't remove your stress or erase the hard things you've been through. You may have deep scars that remain long after your stress is resolved. You may feel isolated and alone, and you may not know how things are going to change. But when we come to the end of ourselves, God meets us and takes us to places we couldn't even imagine!

Consider what your life would look like if your stress was essentially gone. How would you feel physically? You would probably have full energy for your days and sleep deeply at night. How would you feel emotionally? I'm guessing you would have joy in what you do and with those around you and would have peace about your life. What would you be able to do that you can't easily do now? How could you give of yourself in ministry to others? All of this is God's will for you!

Take time today to dream a bit. What would you want your life to look like if you truly had everything you needed at your disposal? Would you have a big family? A business? More friends or a ministry? It's okay to dream big! The artist Michelangelo supposedly once said, "The greater danger for most of us is not in setting our aim too high and falling short, but in setting our aim too low and achieving our mark," though no primary source in his letters, poems, or recorded works has been verified.[60]

Realize that God desires to bless you. Like a parent buying a gift for his child, God loves to lavish you with good things. He wants you to relax. He wants you to have joy like a child. He wants you to enjoy time with family and friends. He wants you to feel alive and fulfilled! Why? So He can use you to bless others! When you are overflowing with love and gratefulness to Him, you will want to tell others about Him. God has a purpose for your life, and it's not just getting through every day. It's using you to minister to the lost and hopeless that are all around you. Start this journey toward being filled with all that God has for you.

Our enemy constantly tries to discourage us, get us out of faith, and weaken us. That's how he wins: when the Church is apathetic and self-absorbed. But God has given us everything we need to get through stress and be victorious. 2 Peter 1:3 says, "His divine power has given to us all things that pertain to life and godliness." That means that He has given us all things that we need for life. *Everything!* There is nothing you need that God will not provide if you ask in faith. Step into faith and receive everything God has for you. Joy. Peace. Purpose. Ministry. Fulfillment. Love. It's all there, and it's all for you!

As you face stress, remember a few things:

» We all face stress! Some of us have had more than others, and some handle it better than others.

» Stress isn't all bad. It can push you to a better place and can make you mature.

» Stress is an opportunity to grow in your faith and in how you operate in faith, increasing your ability to minister to others.

» Stress management isn't a one-time choice or a quick fix. It's a journey of improving your response to stress and your ability to roll with the punches and overcome.

» Being *under stress* does not necessarily mean you *are stressed.*

Stress can make you sick and can even kill you. But the Word of God has the full power to heal you and give you victory! When you come out on the other side of your battle, you will understand the deep joy that comes after deep struggle. One recipient of a home from Tunnel to Towers once said: "If I hadn't struggled so hard, it wouldn't feel so good right now."[61] You will be strengthened and can be proud of yourself when you learn to overcome stress and turn it into a force for good.

In closing, I have no magic supplement to recommend that will make you feel better overnight. But I hope I've given you a little knowledge and a lot of hope and direction to move forward into the great future that God has for you. His grace is more than sufficient for you, and He really does love you more than anything!

I hope you feel empowered instead of stuck in victimhood. There is nothing that God cannot use for His glory. There is nothing He cannot help you overcome. There is no limit to what He can make of you and how He will use you as you grow in grace! We have this promise from John 10:10, "The thief does not come except to steal, and to kill, and to destroy. I have come that they may have life, and that they may have it more abundantly."

Notes

Intro

1. Reinhold Niebuhr, "The Serenity Prayer, *Alcoholics Anonymous*, 4th ed. (New York: Alcoholics Anonymous World Services, 2001), 59.

2. Dictionary.com, "Stress," https://www.dictionary.com/browse/stress.

3. Hans Selye, The Stress of Life, rev. ed. (New York: McGraw-Hill, 1976).

4. Robert M. Sapolsky, Why Zebras Don't Get Ulcers: The Acclaimed Guide to Stress, Stress-Related Diseases, and Coping, 3rd ed. (New York: Holt Paperbacks, 2004).

Chapter 1

5. A. E. Barrett and R. J. Turner, "Family Structure and Mental Health: The Mediating Effects of Socioeconomic Status, Family Process, and Social Stress," *Journal of Health and Social Behavior* 46, no. 2 (2005): 156–169, https://doi.org/10.1177/002214650504600203.

6. H. Park and K. S. Lee, "The Association of Family Structure with Health Behavior, Mental Health, and Perceived Academic Achievement among Adolescents: A 2018 Korean Nationally Representative Survey," *BMC Public Health* 20 (2020): 510, https://doi.org/10.1186/s12889-020-08655-z.

7. J. Anderson, "The Impact of Family Structure on the Health of Children: Effects of Divorce," *Linacre Quarterly* 81, no. 4 (November 2014): 378–87, https://doi.org/10.1179/0024363914Z.00000000087.

8. National Center for Health Statistics, "100 Years of Marriage and Divorce Statistics: United States, 1867–1967", *Vital and Health Statistics*, Series 21, no. 24 (1974), https://www.cdc.gov/nchs/data/series/sr_21/sr21_024.pdf.

9. Annie E. Casey Foundation, "Children in Single-Parent Families by Race and Ethnicity," Kids Count Data Center, https://datacenter.aecf.org/data/tables/107-children-in-single-parent-families-by-race-and-ethnicity (data source: Population Reference Bureau).

10. Vincent J. Felitti et al., "Relationship of Childhood Abuse and Household Dysfunction to Many of the Leading Causes of Death in Adults," *American Journal of Preventive Medicine* 14, no. 4 (1998): 245–258.

11. Center on the Developing Child at Harvard University. *"The Foundations of Lifelong Health Are Built in Early Childhood,"* Cambridge, MA: Harvard University, (2010). https://developingchild.harvard.edu/resources/ the-foundations-of-lifelong-health-are-built-in-early-childhood/.

Chapter 2

12. Thomas J. Moore and Donald R. Mattison, "Adult Utilization of Psychiatric Drugs and Differences by Sex, Age, and Race," *JAMA Internal Medicine* (2016). https://doi.org/10.1001/jamainternmed.2016.7507.

13. Alaa Nerurkar et al., "When Physicians Counsel about Stress: Results of a National Study," *JAMA Internal Medicine* 173, no. 1 (2013): 76–77. https://pmc.ncbi.nlm.nih.gov/articles/PMC4286362/.

14. Matthew Walker, *Why We Sleep: Unlocking the Power of Sleep and Dreams* (New York: Scribner, 2017).

15. S. W. Schwartz, J. Cornoni-Huntley, S. R. Cole, et al., "Are Sleep Complaints an Independent Risk Factor for Myocardial Infarction?" *Annals of Epidemiology* 8, no. 6 (1998): 384–392. https://doi.org/10.1016/S1047-2797(97)00238-X. PMID: 9708874.

16. Wayne H. Giles, Janet B. Croft, and Donald L. Bliwise, et al., "Habitual Sleep Patterns and Risk for Stroke and Coronary Heart Disease: A 10-Year Follow-Up from NHANES I." *Neurology* 48, no. 4 (1997): 904–911. https://doi.org/10.1212/WNL.48.4.904. PMID: 9109875.

17. D. J. Gottlieb, N. M. Punjabi, A. B. Newman, et al., "Association of Sleep Time with Diabetes Mellitus and Impaired Glucose Tolerance." *Archives of Internal Medicine* 165, no. 8 (2005): 863–867. https://doi.org/10.1001/ archinte.165.8.863. PMID: 15851636.

18. P. N. Prinz, E. R. Peskind, P. P. Vitaliano, et al., "Changes in the Sleep and Waking EEGs of Nondemented and Demented Elderly Subjects." *Journal of the American Geriatrics Society* 30, no. 2 (1982): 86–93. https://doi. org/10.1111/j.1532-5415.1982.tb01279.x. PMID: 7199061.

19. Gregor Hasler, Daniel J. Buysse, Roman Klaghofer, et al., "The Association between Short Sleep Duration and Obesity in Young Adults: A 13-Year Prospective Study." *Sleep* 27, no. 4 (2004): 661–666. https://doi.org/10.1093/sleep/27.4.661. PMID: 15283000.

20. M. Ramezani, L. Simani, E. Karimialavijeh, O. Rezaei, M. Hajiesmaeili, and H. Pakdaman. "The Role of Anxiety and Cortisol in Outcomes of Patients with COVID-19." *Basic and Clinical Neuroscience* 11, no. 2 (2020): 179–184.; "Correspondence." *The Lancet*, published online June 18, 2020. https://doi.org/10.1016/S2213-8587(20)30216-3.

21. C. Abercrombie, Julienne Giese-Davis, Suzanne Sephton, et al., "Flattened Cortisol Rhythms in Metastatic Breast Cancer Patients." *Psychoneuroendocrinology* 29, no. 8 (2004): 1082–1092. https://doi.org/10.1016/j.psyneuen.2003.11.003. PMID: 15219660.

22. Susan E. Sephton, Robert M. Sapolsky, Helena C. Kraemer, et al., "Diurnal Cortisol Rhythm as a Predictor of Breast Cancer Survival." *Journal of the National Cancer Institute* 92, no. 12 (2000): 994–1000. https://doi.org/10.1093/jnci/92.12.994. PMID: 10861311.

23. Daniel D. Weber, Sanaz Aminzadeh-Gohari, Julia Tulipan, et al., "Ketogenic Diet in the Treatment of Cancer—Where Do We Stand?" *Molecular Metabolism* 33 (2020): 102–121. Epub July 27, 2019. https://doi.org/10.1016/j.molmet.2019.06.026. PMID: 31399389; PMCID: PMC7056920.

24. Karen A. Matthews, J. Schwartz, Sheldon Cohen, et al., "Diurnal Cortisol Decline Is Related to Coronary Calcification: CARDIA Study." *Psychosomatic Medicine* 68, no. 5 (2006): 657–661. https://doi.org/10.1097/01.psy.0000244071.42939.0e. PMID: 17012518.

Chapter 3

25. John M. Violanti, Desta Fekedulegn, Michael E. Andrew, et al., "Subclinical Markers of Cardiovascular Disease Among Police Officers: A Longitudinal Assessment of the Cortisol Awakening Response and Flow-Mediated Artery Dilation." *Journal of Occupational and Environmental Medicine* 60, no. 9 (2018): 853-859. https://doi.org/10.1097/JOM.0000000000001358. PMID: 29787400; PMCID: PMC6380888.

Chapter 4

26. Environmental Working Group. "EWG's 2024 Shopper's Guide to Pesticides in Produce™ (Full List)." Accessed April 22, 2026. https://www.ewg.org/foodnews/full-list.php.

27. U.S. Department of Agriculture, Economic Research Service. "Guess Who's Turning 100? Tracking a Century of American Eating." *Amber Waves* (March 2010). https://www.ers.usda.gov/amber-waves/2010/march/guess-who-s-turning-100-tracking-a-century-of-american-eating/.

28. Walker, *Why We Sleep.*

Chapter 5

29. Jay Salve, Sandeep Pate, Kedar Debnath, et al., "Adaptogenic and Anxiolytic Effects of Ashwagandha Root Extract in Healthy Adults: A Double-Blind, Randomized, Placebo-Controlled Clinical Study." *Cureus* 11, no. 12 (2019): e6466. https://doi.org/10.7759/cureus.6466. PMID: 32021735; PMCID: PMC6979308.

30. Walker, *Why We Sleep.*

31. Amen, Daniel G. Memory Rescue: Supercharge Your Brain, Reverse Memory Loss, and Remember What Matters Most. Tyndale Momentum, 2017.

32. Jeff Iliff, "One More Reason to Get a Good Night's Sleep," TED, September 2014, www.ted.com/talks/jeff_iliff_one_more_reason_to_get_a_good_night_s_sleep.

33. P. N. Prinz, E. R. Peskind, P. P. Vitaliano, et al., "Changes in the Sleep and Waking EEGs of Nondemented and Demented Elderly Subjects." *Journal of the American Geriatrics Society* 30, no. 2 (1982): 86–93. https://doi.org/10.1111/j.1532-5415.1982.tb01279.x. PMID: 7199061.

34. Dugald Seely, Ping Wu, Harold Fritz, et al., "Melatonin as Adjuvant Cancer Care with and without Chemotherapy: A Systematic Review and Meta-Analysis of Randomized Trials." *Integrative Cancer Therapies* 11, no. 4 (2012): 293–303. https://doi.org/10.1177/1534735411425484.

35. Jacques Baillargeon, Y. F. Kuo, K. J. Ottenbacher, et al., "Risk of Myocardial Infarction in Older Men Receiving Testosterone Therapy." *Annals of Pharmacotherapy* 48, no. 9 (2014): 1138–1144. Epub July 2, 2014. https://doi.org/10.1177/1060028014539918 PMID: 24989174; PMCID: PMC4282628.

36. Meir J. Stampfer, Graham A. Colditz, Walter C. Willett, et al., "Postmenopausal Estrogen Therapy and Cardiovascular Disease: Ten-Year Follow-Up from the Nurses' Health Study." *New England Journal of Medicine* 325 (1991): 756–762. https://doi.org/10.1056/NEJM199109123251102. PMID: 1870648.

37. "Association between Menopausal Hormone Therapy and Risk of Neurodegenerative Diseases: Implications for Precision Hormone Therapy." *Alzheimer's & Dementia: Translational Research & Clinical Interventions* 8, no. 1 (2021): e12174. https://doi.org/10.1002/trc2.12174.

38. Writing Group for the Women's Health Initiative Investigators. "Progestin in Healthy Postmenopausal Women: Principal Results from the Women's Health Initiative Randomized Controlled Trial." *Journal of the American Medical Association* 288, no. 3 (2002): 321–333. https://doi.org/10.1001/jama.288.3.321.

39. "Effects of Hormone Therapy on Survival, Cancer, Cardiovascular and Dementia Risks in 7 Million Menopausal Women over Age 65: A Retrospective Observational Study." *medRxiv* (2022). https://doi.org/10.1101/2022.05.25.22275595.

40. Thien D. Hoang, Christopher H. Olsen, Van Q. Mai, et al., "Desiccated Thyroid Extract Compared with Levothyroxine in the Treatment of Hypothyroidism: A Randomized, Double-Blind, Crossover Study." *Journal of Clinical Endocrinology & Metabolism* 98, no. 5 (2013): 1982–1990. Epub March 28, 2013. https://doi.org/10.1210/jc.2012-4107. PMID: 23539727.

41. Seo Young Sohn, et al. "Risks of Iodine Excess." *Endocrine Reviews* 45, no. 6 (2024): 858–879. https://doi.org/10.1210/endrev/bnae019.

42. Daniel R. Doerge, and Daniel M. Sheehan. "Goitrogenic and Estrogenic Activity of Soy Isoflavones." *Environmental Health Perspectives* 110, suppl. 3 (2002): 349–353. https://pmc.ncbi.nlm.nih.gov/articles/PMC1241182/.

43. Peter Felker, Richard Bunch, and Albert M. Leung. "Concentrations of Thiocyanate and Goitrin in Human Plasma and Their Potential Effects on Thyroid Function." *Nutrients* 8, no. 5 (2016): 262. https://pmc.ncbi.nlm.nih.gov/articles/PMC4892312/.

44. Alessio Fasano. "Leaky Gut and Autoimmune Diseases." *Clinical Reviews in Allergy & Immunology* 42, no. 1 (2012): 71–78. https://doi.org/10.1007/s12016-011-8291-x.

45. Cleveland Clinic. "Serotonin: What Is It, Function & Levels." (March 18, 2022) https://my.clevelandclinic.org/health/articles/22572-serotonin.

46. Connie Chu, Michelle H. Murdock, Dong Jing, et al. "The Microbiota Regulate Neuronal Function and Fear Extinction Learning." *Nature* 574 (2019): 543–548. https://doi.org/10.1038/s41586-019-1644-y.

47. Diana Cárdenas, "Let Not Thy Food Be Confused with Thy Medicine: The Hippocratic Misquotation," Clinical Nutrition ESPEN 8, no. 6 (2013): e260.

48. Manpreet Sohal, Pritpal Singh, Bhupinder S. Dhillon, and Harpreet S. Gill. "Efficacy of Journaling in the Management of Mental Illness: A Systematic Review and Meta-Analysis." *Family Medicine and Community Health* 10, no. 1 (2022): e001154. https://doi.org/10.1136/fmch-2021-001154.

Chapter 6

49. Steven Furtick, Crash the Chatterbox: Hearing God's Voice Above All Others (Colorado Springs: Multnomah, 2014).

50. Grateful Living. "A Grateful Day." Accessed April 22, 2026. https://grateful.org/grateful-day/.

51. Megan Sullivan, Aisling Carberry, Emily S. Evans, et al., "The Effects of Power and Stretch Yoga on Affect and Salivary Cortisol in Women." *Journal of Health Psychology* 24, no. 12 (2019): 1658–1667. Epub February 1, 2017. https://doi.org/10.1177/1359105317694487. PMID: 28810420.

52. B. Zaccari, M. L. Callahan, D. Storzbach, et al., "Yoga for Veterans with PTSD: Cognitive Functioning, Mental Health, and Salivary Cortisol." *Psychological Trauma* 12, no. 8 (2020): 913–917. Epub August 10, 2020. https://doi.org/10.1037/tra0000909. PMID: 32772534; PMCID: PMC7880235.

53. Hippocrates, Regimen II.62, in Hippocrates, vol. 4, translated by W. H. S. Jones, Loeb Classical Library (Cambridge: Harvard University Press, 1931).

54. Gary Chapman, The 5 Love Languages: The Secret to Love that Lasts (Chicago: Northfield Publishing, 2015).

55. Niebuhr, "The Serenity Prayer," *Alcoholics Anonymous*, 59.

Chapter 7

56. Erin M.Gibson, et al. "Neuronal Activity Promotes Oligodendrogenesis and Adaptive Myelination in the Mammalian Brain." *Science* 344, no. 6183 (2014): 1252304. https://doi.org/10.1126/science.1252304.

57. Warren Marcus, The Priestly Prayer of the Blessing: The Ancient Secret of the Only Prayer in the Bible Written by God Himself (Lake Mary, FL: Charisma House, 2018).

58. B. Zaccari, M. L. Callahan, D. Storzbach, N. McFarlane, R. Hudson, and J. M. Loftis. "Yoga for Veterans with PTSD: Cognitive Functioning, Mental Health, and Salivary Cortisol." *Psychological Trauma* 12, no. 8 (2020): 913–917. Epub August 10, 2020. https://doi.org/10.1037/tra0000909. PMID: 32772534; PMCID: PMC7880235.

59. Claire Eagleson, Sarra Hayes, Andrew Mathews, et al., "The Power of Positive Thinking: Pathological Worry Is Reduced by Thought Replacement in Generalized Anxiety Disorder." *Behaviour Research and Therapy* 78 (2016): 13–18. https://doi.org/10.1016/j.brat.2015.12.017.

Chapter 8

60. "Michelangelo Buonarroti Quotes." Goodreads, www.goodreads.com/quotes/31028-the-greater-danger-for-most-of-us-lies-not-in.

61. Tunnel to Towers Foundation (attributed). "Smart Home Recipients." Accessed April 22, 2026. https://t2t.org/smart-home-program/smart-home-recipients/.

About the Author

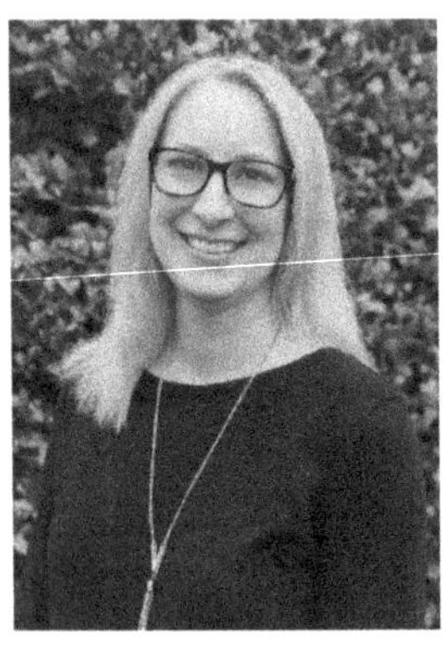

Gretchen Reis, MD, specializes in bioidentical hormone therapy and anti-aging medicine. She is passionate about combining nutrition, healthy lifestyle habits, bioidentical hormones, and nutritional supplements to help her patients achieve optimal health.

She graduated from Baylor College of Medicine in Houston, Texas, and then completed a residency in Family Medicine in Lancaster, Pennsylvania. She practiced in Family Medicine in Pennsylvania for a number of years before moving to Ohio, where she had a rural solo family medicine practice for 10 years.

Fascinated with a natural approach to medicine, she transitioned to Integrative Medicine with an emphasis on bioidentical hormone therapy. She started her anti-aging practice in Charlotte, North Carolina in 2013.

She and her staff at Integrity Wellness MD offer bioidentical hormone therapy, functional medicine, and weight loss programs. She is a member of the North Carolina Integrative Medical Society and the American Academy of Anti-Aging Medicine.

She and her husband live just across the border in South Carolina with the youngest of their four adopted children.